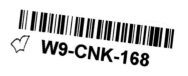

Interventional Cardiology
The Essentials for the Boards
Questions and Answers, Clinical Cases and Pearls

Cindy L. Grines, MD
Director
Cardiac Catheterization Laboratories
William Beaumont Hospital
Royal Oak, Michigan

Mihaela A. Savu, MD
Interventional Cardiologist
St. Vincent Infirmary
Baptist Medical Center
Heart Hospital
Little Rock, Arkansas

and

Luis A. Tejada, MD
Interventional Cardiologist
St. Luke's Hospital
Bethlehem, Pennsylvania

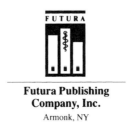

Futura Publishing Company, Inc.
Armonk, NY

Library of Congress Cataloging-in-Publication Data

Grines, Cindy.
   Interventional cardiology : the essentials for the boards :
questions and answers, clinical cases, and pearls / Cindy L.
Grines, Mihaela A. Savu, and Luis Tejada.
      p.   cm.
   Includes bibliographical references.
   ISBN 0-87993-443-3 (alk. paper)
   1. Heart—Diseases—Treatment Examinations, questions,
etc.   2. Cardiovascular system—Diseases—Treatment
Examinations, questions, etc.   I. Savu, Mihaela A.
II. Tejada, Luis, M.D.   III. Title.
   [DNLM: 1. Cardiovascular Diseases—diagnosis
Examination Questions.   WG 18.2 G866i 1999]
RC683.8.G75 1999
616.1′2—dc21
DNLM/DLC
   for Library of Congress   99–27741
                                                              CIP

Copyright © 1999
Futura Publishing Company, Inc.

Published by
Futura Publishing Company, Inc.
135 Bedford Road
Armonk, New York 10504-0418

ISBN #: 0-87993-443-3

Every effort has been made to ensure that the information in this book is as up to date and as accurate as possible at the time of publication. However, due to the constant developments in medicine, neither the author, nor the editor, nor the publisher can accept any legal or any other responsibility for any errors or omissions that may occur.

Printed in the United States of America.

This book is printed on acid-free paper.

Dedication

To my husband, Calin, and my parents, Ivona and Mitus,
for their unconditional love
M.S.

To my husband Doug and son John,
for their love and support,
to my son, Derek, for preventing progress
by losing every tape recorder in the Cardiology Division,
and to my daughter, Jessica,
for causing so little trouble as a teen
that I could accomplish this project!
C.L.G.

To my parents, for their love and support
L.A.T.

Contents

Chapter 1

Anatomy and Physiology

QUESTIONS

1.   Of the following statements regarding coronary spasm, all are TRUE, **EXCEPT:**

    a.   Coronary artery spasm has been reported in 1% to 5% of balloon angioplasty procedures.
    b.   Variant angina does not predict procedure-related spasm.
    c.   Spontaneous episodes of spasm may develop months following percutaneous transluminal coronary angioplasty (PTCA) and may cause angina.
    d.   One of the mechanisms of side-branch occlusion is coronary spasm.
    e.   Repeat balloon inflation at the involved site is contraindicated, as it may worsen the spasm.

2.   How do you define "severely angulated" lesion?

    a.   Lesion associated with 45° to 90° bend.
    b.   Lesion associated with more than 90° bend.
    c.   Lesion associated with two bends.
    d.   Lesion associated with more than two 45° bends.

Using the NHLBI Registry scoring system, match the following types of coronary dissections with the corresponding definition:

3.   Double lumen separated by a radiolucent area during contrast injections with minimal persistence after dye clearance.

4.   Contrast material seen immediately outside the coronary lumen but within the vessel wall.

5.   Linear radiolucent area within the coronary lumen with minimal persistence of contrast dye.

6.   Spiral luminal filling defects with contrast material staining of the vessel.

7.   Total occlusion.

    a. Type A
    b. Type B
    c. Type C
    d. Type D
    e. Type E
    f. Type F

8.   A 60-year-old man is referred to you for rescue angioplasty. In the cardiac catheterization laboratory, the patient has 7/10 chest pain; he denies other symptoms. His blood pressure (BP) is 130/70 mm Hg and his heart rate (HR) is 82 bpm, in sinus rhythm. An 8F plasty sheath is placed in the right femoral artery over the wire. The angiography reveals a total occlusion of mid right coronary artery (RCA). The first balloon inflation successfully reestablishes thrombolysis in myocardial infarction (TIMI) grade 2-3 flow. At this time patient complains of dizziness and his systolic BP drops to 60 mm Hg, and his HR to 38 bpm, in sinus bradycardia.

What is the most likely explanation for this acute problem?

    a. Patient developed cardiac tamponade.
    b. This is a reperfusion-related event.
    c. Patient has an acute bleeding due to recent use of thrombolytic therapy.
    d. This is a delayed vasovagal episode related to sheath insertion.

9.   Of the following statements regarding the coronary ectasia, all are TRUE, **EXCEPT:**

    a. The underlying histologic changes are identical to those found in atherosclerotic lesions.
    b. Coronary artery ectasia is a benign finding.
    c. Prognosis of patients with coronary ectasia is better than the prognosis of patients with critically stenotic coronaries.

    d. A possible relationship exists between coronary ectasia and herbicides.

10. Of the following statements regarding coronary blood flow, all are TRUE, **EXCEPT:**

    a. Fractional flow reserves (FFRs) are easy to measure, but differ with hemodynamic changes.
    b. Small vessel disease can be detected by using Doppler flow wire.
    c. Coronary flow reserve (CFR) is defined as the ratio of hyperemic blood flow to baseline blood flow.
    d. Left ventricular hypertrophy may spuriously decrease the CFR.

11. Of the following statements regarding intracoronary pressure measurements, all are TRUE, **EXCEPT:**

    a. They can be obtained with a fiberoptic wire capable of detecting changes in reflected light from a mirror source deformed by pressure changes.
    b. They can be obtained with a fluid-filled wire.
    c. FFR of the myocardium (FFRmyo) can be obtained.
    d. Intracoronary pressure measurements have prognostic implications.

12. Of the following statements regarding the ankle-brachial index (ABI), all are TRUE, **EXCEPT:**

    a. It is a marker of diffuse atherosclerosis when it is ≤0.9.
    b. It localizes the area of stenosis or occlusion.
    c. It can stratify a patient's risk of wound healing and the development of ischemic rest pain.
    d. It can be worsened with an exercise treadmill stress test.

13. Of the following statements regarding cardiac metabolic regulation, all are TRUE, **EXCEPT:**

    a. Baseline coronary venous oxygen saturation is 25% to 30%.

b. Adenosine is a mediator that links metabolically induced vasodilatation to diminished coronary perfusion.
c. Coronary reactive hyperemia defines the increase in
coronary blood flow above the baseline immediately after the flow is reestablished in a temporarily occluded
artery.
d. Myocardium depends entirely on anaerobic metabolism.

14.   Which one of the following drugs needs an intact endothelium in order to produce vasodilatation?

a. Nitroglycerin
b. Acetylcholine
c. Prostacyclin (PGI$_2$)
d. Adenosine

15.   Of the following statements regarding the ankle-brachial
systolic index (ABSI), all are TRUE, **EXCEPT:**

a. If the patient has intermittent claudication and the index is above 0.8 at rest and above 0.5 after 5 minutes of
exercise, the arterial insufficiency is mild.
b. Brachial systolic pressure is measured in both arms
and the higher value is used to calculate right and left
indexes.
c. Claudication, ABSI <0.5 before exercise, and <0.15 after exercise are markers of severe arterial insufficiency.
d. The ABSI is especially useful for confirmation and estimation of the degree of functional impairment in diabetics.

16.   To which anatomical zone does the deep femoral artery
belong?

a. Inflow tract
b. Outflow tract
c. Run-off bed

ANSWERS

1. Of the following statements regarding coronary spasm, all are TRUE, **EXCEPT:**

    a. Coronary artery spasm has been reported in 1% to 5% of balloon angioplasty procedures.
    b. Variant angina does not predict procedure-related spasm.
    c. Spontaneous episodes of spasm may develop months following percutaneous transluminal coronary angioplasty (PTCA) and may cause angina.
    d. One of the mechanisms of side-branch occlusion is coronary spasm.
    e. Repeat balloon inflation at the involved site is contraindicated, as it may worsen the spasm.

ANSWER: e

Coronary artery spasm has been reported in 1% to 5% of balloon angioplasty procedures. Risk factors include:

- noncalcified lesions
- possibly eccentric lesions
- younger patients

but not variant angina (*J Am Coll Cardiol* 1985;5:1046–1054).

Prolonged low-pressure inflation with a size-matched balloon is useful when nitrates intracoronary (I.C.) have failed. Perfusion balloons should be used for refractory spasm. As a last resort, coronary stenting can be considered.

Most commonly, side-branch occlusion occurs because of "snow plow" effect, but other mechanisms include spasm (more often during atherectomy and laser procedures), propagating dissection originating in the parent vessel, and distal embolization.

Beware of "pseudolesions," which occur on bend points and are due to straightening or torsion of a bend point with a stiff guidewire. These lesions resolve with removal of the wire or exchange for a floppy wire.

2. How do you define "severely angulated" lesion?

    a. Lesion associated with 45° to 90° bend.
    b. Lesion associated with more than 90° bend.

c.   Lesion associated with two bends.
d.   Lesion associated with more than two 45° bends.

ANSWER: b

Lesions associated with bends of 45° to 90° are simply classified as "angulated," and lesions with bends of 90° or more are commonly classified as "severely angulated." Lesion angulation should be assessed in a nonforeshortened end-diastolic projection (Braunwald E. *Heart Disease: A Textbook of Cardiovascular Medicine*. Philadelphia: W.B. Saunders Co.; 1997:265).

Using the NHLBI Registry scoring system, match the following types of coronary dissections with the corresponding definition:

3.   Double lumen separated by a radiolucent area during contrast injections with minimal persistence after dye clearance.

4.   Contrast material seen immediately outside the coronary lumen but within the vessel wall.

5.   Linear radiolucent area within the coronary lumen with minimal persistence of contrast dye.

6.   Spiral luminal filling defects with contrast material staining of the vessel.

7.   Total occlusion.

a.   Type A
b.   Type B
c.   Type C
d.   Type D
e.   Type E
f.   Type F

ANSWERS: 3-b, 4-c, 5-a, 6-d, 7-f

The National Heart, Lung, and Blood Institute classification system of intimal dissections is based on angiographic appearance and is graded as follows:

Types A and B dissections are associated with clinical success (93%) as opposed to complex dissections (*types C through F*), which are associated with a low success rate (37%) and a high in-hospital complication rate (these data reflect the pre-stent era [*Am J Cardiol* 1991;68:467–471]).

The *type E* dissection, the single one not defined above, represents new, persistent filling defects (basically indistinguishable from thrombus).

8.   A 60-year-old man is referred to you for rescue angioplasty. In the cardiac catheterization laboratory, the patient has 7/10 chest pain; he denies other symptoms. His blood pressure (BP) is 130/70 mm Hg and his heart rate (HR) is 82 bpm, in sinus rhythm. An 8F plasty sheath is placed in the right femoral artery over the wire. The angiography reveals a total occlusion of mid right coronary artery (RCA). The first balloon inflation successfully reestablishes thrombolysis in myocardial infarction (TIMI) grade II-III flow. At this time patient complains of dizziness and his systolic BP drops to 60 mm Hg, and his HR to 38 bpm, in sinus bradycardia.

What is the most likely explanation for this acute problem?

    a.   Patient developed cardiac tamponade.
    b.   This is a reperfusion-related event.
    c.   Patient has an acute bleeding due to recent use of thrombolytic therapy.
    d.   This is a delayed vasovagal episode related to sheath insertion.

ANSWER: b

This clinical picture is due to Bezold-Jarisch reflex, which should be anticipated by the interventional cardiologist. The usual scenario is that of a patient with ongoing inferior wall myocardial infarction (MI) due to a totally occluded RCA. The patient is otherwise stable hemodynamically until immediately after the flow is reestablished. With reperfusion of RCA, occasional profound hypotension and bradycardia may ensue rapidly. The treatment encompasses repeated doses of atropine, dopamine, intravenous (I.V.) fluids, and, rarely, small amounts of short-acting vasopressors (metaraminol, neosynephrine) (*J Am Coll Cardiol* 1989;14: 1202–1209).

Slow reperfusion with the wire alone, while waiting for reperfusion arrhythmias to resolve, or "dottering" with a deflated balloon, may resolve the incidence of Bezold-Jarisch reflex.

The clinical presentation of acute bleeding or tamponade would include tachycardia, chest pain, and a less sudden onset.

9.   Of the following statements regarding the coronary ectasia, all are TRUE, **EXCEPT:**

    a.   The underlying histologic changes are identical to those found in atherosclerotic lesions.
    b.   Coronary artery ectasia is a benign finding.
    c.   Prognosis of patients with coronary ectasia is better than the prognosis of patients with critically stenotic coronaries.
    d.   A possible relationship exists between coronary ectasia and herbicides.

ANSWER: b

Coronary ectasia is not a benign feature. It predisposes the vessel to spasm, thrombus formation, and spontaneous dissection. The histologic appearance itself is similar to that of atherosclerosis: intimal and medial damage and diffuse hyalinization (*Br Heart J* 1978;40:393–400). Although medial disruption prevents coronary spasm in ectatic vessels, this type of coronary anatomy is predisposed to spasm (in the normal vessel adjacent to the dilated portion) (*Cathet Cardiovasc Diagn* 1994;32:1–7).

The prognosis for patients with coronary ectasia is better than that for patients with coronary stenoses, but worse than for people with normal coronaries.

A potential relationship is possible between chronic exposure to herbicides (containing acetylcholine, which is a stimulant of nitric oxide [NO]) and coronary ectasia (*Med J Aust* 1981;68:260).

10.   Of the following statements regarding coronary blood flow, all are TRUE, **EXCEPT:**

    a.   Fractional flow reserves (FFRs) are easy to measure, but differ with hemodynamic changes.
    b.   Small vessel disease can be detected by using Doppler flow wire.
    c.   Coronary flow reserve (CFR) is defined as the ratio of hyperemic blood flow to baseline blood flow.
    d.   Left ventricular hypertrophy may spuriously decrease the CFR.

ANSWER: a

FFR, defined as the ratio of maximum flow in the presence of a stenosis to normal maximum flow, is a lesion-specific index of stenosis severity. FFR is independent of hemodynamic changes.

Coronary flow velocity reserve (CFVR) is influenced by hemodynamic changes (*Circulation* 1997;96:2094–2095).

CFR, defined as the ratio of hyperemic blood flow to resting blood flow, decreases in the presence of small vessel disease and significant epicardial artery stenosis. The normal CFR measured in humans undergoing catheterization is greater than 2.5.

Different factors can spuriously decrease CFR (ventricular hypertrophy, hypertension).

11.   Of the following statements regarding intracoronary pressure measurements, all are TRUE, **EXCEPT:**

   a. They can be obtained with a fiberoptic wire capable of detecting changes in reflected light from a mirror source deformed by pressure changes.
   b. They can be obtained with a fluid-filled wire.
   c. FFR of the myocardium (FFRmyo) can be obtained.
   d. Intracoronary pressure measurements have prognostic implications.

ANSWER: d

Unlike myocardial perfusion imaging and stress testing, intracoronary pressure measurements have not yet produced long-term prognostic information. In addition, they do not account for stress-induced paradoxical vasoconstriction that may occur in patients with coronary atherosclerosis.

Two angioplasty guidewires have been developed for intracoronary pressure measurements. The Pressure Guide (Radi Medical Systems, Uppsala, Sweden) uses fiberoptics and is relatively stiff. The fluid-filled (Schneider, Bulach, Switzerland) can be connected to any pressure transducer.

FFRmyo is the ratio of maximal hyperemic flow in the stenotic artery to the theoretical maximal hyperemic flow in the same artery without a stenosis. It is computed as the ratio of distal mean pressure and mean aortic pressure during maximal hyperemia, and it has an unequivocal value of 1.0 for every patient.

FFRmyo is generally unaffected by changes in HR, BP, and contractility. An FFRmyo of 0.75 reliably distinguishes a significant stenosis (*J Am Coll Cardiol* 1997;30:613–620).

12.   Of the following statements regarding the ankle-brachial index (ABI), all are TRUE, **EXCEPT:**

    a.   It is a marker of diffuse atherosclerosis when it is ≤0.9.
    b.   It localizes the area of stenosis or occlusion.
    c.   It can stratify a patient's risk of wound healing and the development of ischemic rest pain.
    d.   It can be worsened with an exercise treadmill stress test.

ANSWER: b

ABI does not localize, but measures well the severity of lower extremity atherosclerosis.

ABI of less than 0.9 has been correlated with diffuse atherosclerosis, cardiovascular risk, and overall survival (*Angiology* 1995;46: 211–219).

An ABI of ≤0.6 is associated with multiple segment disease.

Resting ankle pressure of less than 40 mm Hg, toe pressure of less than 30 mm Hg, and an ABI of ≤0.30 are associated with ischemic rest pain.

An ABI of ≤0.15 is associated with multiple-segment total occlusions and impending tissue loss.

Patients with mild claudication have ankle pressures after exercise of less than 50 mm Hg but more than 25 mm Hg lower than brachial pressures.

13.   Of the following statements regarding cardiac metabolic regulation, all are TRUE, **EXCEPT:**

    a.   Baseline coronary venous oxygen saturation is 25% to 30%.
    b.   Adenosine is a mediator that links metabolically induced vasodilatation to diminished coronary perfusion.
    c.   Coronary reactive hyperemia defines the increase in coronary blood flow above the baseline immediately after the flow is reestablished in a temporarily occluded artery.
    d.   Myocardium depends entirely on anaerobic metabolism.

ANSWER: d

The epicardial arteries are conductance vessels, and oppose minimal resistance to coronary blood flow.

Precapillary sphincters have a regulatory function according to the metabolic needs of the myocardium.

Myocardium depends entirely on aerobic metabolism; the oxygen saturation in coronary veins is low (25% to 30%).

14.   Which one of the following drugs needs an intact endothelium in order to produce vasodilatation?

    a. Nitroglycerin
    b. Acetylcholine
    c. Prostacyclin (PGI_2)
    d. Adenosine

ANSWER: b

Acetylcholine will produce vasodilatation only if the endothelium is intact. If the endothelium is not intact, only vasoconstriction will be produced by acetylcholine. Therefore, acetylcholine has an indirect (vasodilator) effect on the vessel, mediated by intact endothelium, and a direct (vasoconstrictor) effect; in normal arteries the vasodilator effect predominates.

An abnormal vasomotor response to acetylcholine suggests endothelial dysfunction (as seen in atherosclerosis).

The very few agents that can produce vasodilatation in the absence of the endothelium, directly on vascular smooth muscle, are adenosine, nitrates, and PGI_2.

15.   Of the following statements regarding the ankle-brachial systolic index (ABSI), all are TRUE, **EXCEPT:**

    a. If the patient has intermittent claudication and the index is above 0.8 at rest and above 0.5 after 5 minutes of exercise, the arterial insufficiency is mild.
    b. Brachial systolic pressure is measured in both arms and the higher value is used to calculate right and left indexes.
    c. Claudication, ABSI <0.5 before exercise, and <0.15 after exercise are markers of severe arterial insufficiency.
    d. The ABSI is especially useful for confirmation and estimation of the degree of functional impairment in diabetics.

ANSWER: d

The ABSI is measured in supine position, before and after exercise (walking on the treadmill at 10% grade, at 1 to 2 mph for up to 5 minutes).

Because of medial calcinosis, which quite often is associated with diabetes mellitus, the systolic ankle pressure may be falsely elevated, and therefore the index is not always valid.

16.   To which anatomical zone does the deep femoral artery belong?

   a. Inflow tract
   b. Outflow tract
   c. Run-off bed

ANSWER: b

Arterial circulation of the lower extremity is divided into:

   I. Inflow tract (zone 1)
        Abdominal aorta
        Iliac arteries (common, external, and internal)
   II. Outflow tract (zone 2)
        Femoral arteries (common, deep, and
        superficial)
   III. Run-off bed (zone 3)
        Tibio-peroneal trunk
        Tibial arteries (anterior and posterior)
        Peroneal artery
        Dorsalis pedis

Chapter 2

Pathophysiology

QUESTIONS

1.   It is known that the following cardiovascular risk factors are associated with endothelial dysfunction. Which of the following is **NOT** associated with both impaired NO activity and high endothelin levels?

    a. Hypercholesterolemia
    b. Hypertension
    c. Vascular aging
    d. Diabetes
    e. Estrogen deficiency

2.   Which one of the following statements regarding PGI_2 is TRUE?

    a. It increases cyclic 3′,5′-guanosine monophosphate (cGMP) in smooth muscle and platelets.
    b. It is released by platelets as a response to hypoxia.
    c. It does not contribute to endothelium-dependent relaxation.
    d. It inhibits platelet aggregation.

3.   Clinical and pathologic studies have confirmed that disruption or superficial erosion of atherosclerotic plaque is the major cause of coronary thrombosis. Of the following statements regarding the plaque disruption, all are TRUE, **EXCEPT:**

    a. Loss of collagen matrix represents a critical step toward plaque disruption.
    b. The main thrombogenic components of the plaque are the lipid core and the collagen.
    c. Plaque disruption is frequently asymptomatic and the associated rapid plaque growth is often clinically silent.
    d. Ten percent of all acute MIs are associated with "trigger" activities.

4.   Which of the following statements best describes the pathogenesis of restenosis?

    a. Neointimal hyperplasia is maximal at 2 to 4 months after initial vascular injury.

b. Arterial remodeling (ie, change in vessel size) plays a major role in restenosis.
c. Endothelial regeneration starts in the center of the denuded area, where the vascular injury was maximal, and spreads centrifugally until the endothelial continuity is reestablished.
d. There is evidence that previous restenosis is a risk factor for restenosis.

5.   Of the following statements regarding arterial remodeling after angioplasty, all are TRUE, **EXCEPT:**

a. Restenosis after angioplasty is a balance between intimal formation and arterial remodeling.
b. Arterial remodeling is described in de novo atherosclerosis as well as post angioplasty.
c. Arterial remodeling is defined as constriction or "shrinkage" of the vessel with loss in coronary diameter after coronary intervention.
d. Stents basically eliminate arterial remodeling.

6.   Of the following statements regarding late lumen loss, all are TRUE, **EXCEPT:**

a. It represents the difference between the lumen diameter after the intervention and at 6 months' follow-up.
b. It reflects the net effects of intimal hyperplasia (IH), elastic recoil, and vascular remodeling.
c. Late loss averages 0.5 mm for PTCA and 0.9 mm for stents.
d. The relationship between acute gain and late loss is constant among devices.

7.   Of the following statements regarding aorto-coronary saphenous vein graft (SVG) disease, all are TRUE, **EXCEPT:**

a. During the first year up to 15% of grafts occlude, between 1 and 6 years the attrition rate is 1% to 2% per year, and between 6 and 10 years it is 4% per year.

b. Between 3% and 12% of grafts occlude within the first month, usually due to thrombosis.

c. IH is the major disease process between 1 month and 1 year.

d. Atherosclerosis is the dominant process beyond the first year; this is rarely significant before the third year.

e. Severity of native disease proximal to the anastomosis does not influence SVG disease.

8. Of the following statements regarding acute vessel closure post PTCA, all are TRUE, **EXCEPT:**

a. Approximately half of these will occur immediately postballoon inflation, and they are successfully treated with stents in more than 90% of cases.

b. Up to 10% of late acute closures may not develop electrocardiographic (ECG) changes, especially if the intervention was performed in the circumflex artery or if there were well developed collaterals.

c. The incidence of acute closure is around 15% of all interventions.

d. Risk factors associated with death after acute closure include female gender, large ischemic burden, left ventricular function <30%, and proximal RCA PTCA.

9. Of the following statements about vascular access complications, all are TRUE, **EXCEPT:**

a. Surgical repair is required in 0.9% to 3.5% of all procedures.

b. Risk factors include preprocedural thrombolytic therapy, anticoagulation with warfarin, long-term use of corticosteroids, peripheral vascular disease, and female gender.

c. Ultrasonography-guided compression of a pseudoaneurysm is successful in only 50% of cases.

d. Early sheath removal, smaller diameter arterial sheaths, mechanical, or pneumatic compression devices may reduce vascular complications.

10.   Which one of the following is NOT a risk factors for contrast-induced nephropathy?

    a. Preexisting renal dysfunction
    b. Amount but not type of contrast agent
    c. Diabetes mellitus
    d. Second dose of contrast within 72 hours
    e. Concomitant therapy with nonsteroidal anti-inflammatory agents

11.   Of the following statements regarding cholesterol embolization, all are TRUE, **EXCEPT:**

    a. It is due to microembolism of cholesterol crystals and other atherosclerotic debris after catheter manipulation resulting in occlusion of distal medium sized arteries.
    b. Laboratory test results include eosinophilia, eosinophiluria, elevated sedimentation rate, and decreased complement levels.
    c. Cutaneous manifestations include livedo reticularis, gangrene, and acrocyanosis.
    d. Nervous system manifestations include transient ischemic attacks, amaurosis fugax, and cranial and ocular paralysis.
    e. The triad of leg/foot pain, livedo reticularis, and intact peripheral pulses is considered pathognomonic.

12.   All of the following are predictors of restenosis after stent implantation, **EXCEPT:**

    a. Not using IVUS
    b. Diabetes mellitus
    c. Multiple stents
    d. Minimal lumen diameter immediately post stenting
    e. Aorto-ostial lesions

Match the following:

13.   Restenosis

14.   Recoil

15.   Remodeling

16.   Compensatory enlargement

  a. Local variation in arterial dimensions within the first minutes of angioplasty.
  b. A change in arterial caliber after coronary interventions.
  c. Lumen stenosis delay as lesion area increases.
  d. Local vascular response to wound healing associated with inevitable injury of balloon angioplasty.

17.   Of the following statements regarding myocardial cell death, all are TRUE, **EXCEPT:**

  a. During myocardial ischemia, myocardial cell metabolism becomes anaerobic and, consequently, myocardial cell hydrogen (H^+) concentration increases.
  b. During myocardial ischemia, there is a decrease in intracellular calcium (Ca^{++}).
  c. During reperfusion, more Ca^{++} enters the cell.
  d. Inhibition of the sodium/hydrogen (Na^+/H^+) exchange system would theoretically prevent or limit cell death.

Match the following:

18.   Modest reduction in the coronary blood flow and reduction of myocardial energy metabolism in a steady state, which may last months.

19.   Normal or high coronary flow and normal or excessive myocardial energy metabolism, lasting hours or days.

20.   Severely reduced coronary blood flow and increasingly reduced myocardial energy metabolism, lasting minutes to hours.

21.   Multiple short attacks of reduced coronary flow followed by complete reperfusion.

    a. Preconditioning
    b. True ischemia
    c. Stunning
    d. Hibernation

22.   Of the following statements regarding the vascular response to stenting, all are TRUE, **EXCEPT:**

    a. Preventing thrombus formation will affect late events.
    b. There are 4 distinct phases of vascular repair after stent-induced injury.
    c. There is a linear relationship between the number of monocytes per artery and the extent of arterial intimal growth.
    d. Insertion of a stent limits elastic recoil but not remodeling.

Match the following:

23.   NO

24.   Metalloproteinase

25.   Endothelin

    a. Increases the vulnerability of fibrous cap.
    b. Modulates coronary autoregulation.
    c. Plasma concentration is elevated in atherosclerosis, congestive heart failure (CHF) and acute MI.

26.   The two factors that passivate platelets at the endothelial level are:

    a. Prostaglandin I-2 and NO
    b. Endothelium-derived relaxing factor and NO
    c. Prostaglandin I-2 and PGI_2

Match the following:

27.   Activated partial thromboplastin time (aPTT)

28. Prothrombin time (PT)

29. Vitamin K

30. Protein C, Protein S

    a. Intrinsic pathway
    b. Anticoagulants
    c. Extrinsic pathway
    d. Platelet membrane glycoproteins
    e. g-Carboxylation of glutamic acid residues

Match the following:

31. Unstable angina

32. Non Q wave MI

33. Transmural MI

    a. White thrombus
    b. Red thrombus

34. Of the following statements regarding the comparison between SVGs and internal mammary artery (IMA) conduits, all are TRUE, **EXCEPT:**

    a. Accelerated atherosclerosis appears commonly in SVGs but is uncommon in IMA conduits.
    b. The internal elastic lamina of IMA is uniform and the media has metabolic supply from the lumen and from vasa vasorum.
    c. IMA diameter more frequently matches the bypassed artery diameter.
    d. The vasodilatatory response is more pronounced in SVGs.

35. During rotational atherectomy, platelet aggregation is:

    a. Not affected

    b. Dependent on burr diameter
    c. Dependent on burr speed

36.   Microcavitation is associated with which one of the following atherectomy devices?

    a. Rotablation
    b. Transluminal extraction catheter (TEC)
    c. Excimer laser
    d. Endoluminal radiation using iridium

37.   Intimal dissection after balloon angioplasty is associated with increased risk of:

    a. Restenosis
    b. Restenosis and acute closure
    c. Acute closure
    d. None of the above

38.   Of the following statements regarding reperfusion therapy for acute MI, all are TRUE, **EXCEPT:**

    a. Thrombolytic therapy is associated with recurrent ischemia in 15% to 30% of cases.
    b. PTCA is associated with better immediate patency rates.
    c. PTCA offers better survival in high-risk patients.
    d. Patients who received thrombolytic therapy should undergo angiography before discharge to define coronary anatomy and need for revascularization.

ANSWERS

1.   It is known that the following cardiovascular risk factors are associated with endothelial dysfunction. Which of the following is **NOT** associated with both impaired NO activity and high endothelin levels?

  a. Hypercholesterolemia
  b. Hypertension
  c. Vascular aging
  d. Diabetes
  e. Estrogen deficiency

ANSWER: b

Hypercholesterolemia inhibits endothelium-dependent relaxation. Oxidized low-density lipoprotein (LDL) impairs the activity of NO synthase. Under the conditions of both hypercholesterolemia and atherosclerosis, biologically active NO is markedly reduced and endothelial cell production of endothelin is increased. Plasma levels of endothelin correlate positively with the extent of atherosclerotic lesion formation.

In salt-induced hypertension there is marked impairment of endothelial NO synthase activity. In genetic hypertension the activity of enzyme NO synthase is markedly increased but inefficacious, probably due to increased inactivation of NO by superoxide anion. Plasma levels of endothelin remain normal in most patients with hypertension, except in the presence of renal failure or atherosclerosis.

Vascular aging is associated with a decrease in basal and stimulated release of NO and with reduced expression of the endothelial NO synthase gene. Plasma levels of endothelin increase with aging, but the response to endothelin decreases.

Diabetes is associated with increased levels of endothelin and impairment of the L-arginine-NO pathway.

Estrogen modulates NO synthase activity and the formation of NO. Estrogen deficiency is associated with high levels of circulating endothelin. Endothelin can be inhibited by estrogen in vitro and in vivo (*Clin Cardiol* 1997;20[suppl II]:II3-II10).

2.   Which one of the following statements regarding PGI$_2$ is TRUE?

    a. It increases cyclic 3',5'-guanosine monophosphate (cGMP) in smooth muscle and platelets.
    b. It is released by platelets as a response to hypoxia.
    c. It does not contribute to endothelium-dependent relaxation.
    d. It inhibits platelet aggregation.

ANSWER: d

In addition to NO, endothelial cells release PGI$_2$ in response to shear stresses, hypoxia, and several substances (Ach, 5-HT) that also release NO.

PGI$_2$ increases cyclic 3',5'-adenosine monophosphate (cAMP) in smooth muscle and platelets. Its platelet-inhibitory effects play a greater physiologic role than its contribution to endothelium-dependent relaxation. NO and PGI$_2$ synergistically inhibit platelet aggregation, suggesting that the presence of both mediators is required for maximal inhibition of platelet activation.

3.   Clinical and pathologic studies have confirmed that disruption or superficial erosion of atherosclerotic plaque is the major cause of coronary thrombosis. Of the following statements regarding the plaque disruption, all are TRUE, **EXCEPT:**

    a. Loss of collagen matrix represents a critical step toward plaque disruption.
    b. The main thrombogenic components of the plaque are the lipid core and the collagen.
    c. Plaque disruption is frequently asymptomatic and the associated rapid plaque growth is often clinically silent.
    d. Ten percent of all acute MIs are associated with "trigger" activities.

ANSWER: d

Mature atherosclerotic plaques are composed of two main components: a lipid-rich core and an extracellular matrix. Loss of collagen matrix could result from excessive matrix degradation or reduced matrix synthesis. Macrophages and, to a lesser extent, foam cells derived from smooth muscle cell in atherosclerotic plaques produce a family of matrix-degrading metalloproteinases that are capable of degrading virtually all components of the extracellular matrix.

The main thrombogenic components of the plaque are the lipid core and the collagen. The greater thrombogenicity of the lipid core may be due to its high content of catalytically active factor, a procoagulant transmembrane glycoprotein produced mostly by macrophages in the atherosclerotic plaque. When exposed to circulating blood, tissue factor interacts with factor VIIa and forms a complex that activates factor X. Activated factor Xa initiates the thrombogenic cascade by cleaving prothrombin to thrombin, which, in turn, triggers the coagulation and platelet activation that results in thrombus formation.

Autopsy studies have shown that 9% of healthy persons and up to 22% of diabetic and hypertensive patients have asymptomatic disrupted plaques in their coronary arteries. Coronary occlusion does not necessarily have to progress to MI if there is adequate collateral circulation at the time of the occlusion. Nonetheless, plaque disruption, followed by variable degrees of hemorrhage into the plaque as well as luminal thrombosis, may accelerate further plaque growth and the progression of stenosis, thus accounting for the sudden, nonlinear, and unpredictable progression of coronary atherosclerosis to acute coronary syndromes.

At least half of all acute MIs are associated with "trigger" activities or conditions, which are referred to as *acute risk factors*. These risk factors include vigorous exercise (especially in deconditioned individuals), emotional stress, earthquake, cold weather, time of the day (ie, early morning), and day of the week (ie, Mondays) (*J Am Coll Cardiol* 1994;23:809–813), (*Am J Cardiol* 1990;66:22–27), (*N Engl J Med* 1993;329:1684–1690).

4.   Which of the following statements best describes the pathogenesis of restenosis?

   a. Neointimal hyperplasia is maximal at 2 to 4 months after initial vascular injury.
   b. Arterial remodeling (ie, change in vessel size) plays a major role in restenosis.
   c. Endothelial regeneration starts in the center of the denuded area, where the vascular injury was maximal, and spreads centrifugally until the endothelial continuity is reestablished.
   d. There is evidence that previous restenosis is a risk factor for restenosis.

ANSWER: b

Restenosis after PTCA is a complex process consisting of a combination of elastic recoil, intimal thickening, and vascular remodeling.

Most elastic recoil occurs in the first 30 minutes after balloon deflation (but may occur up to 24 hours) and is more common after PTCA of eccentric and ostial lesions. Elastic recoil is greatest after PTCA, intermediate after directional coronary atherectomy (DCA), and lowest after stenting. Elimination of elastic recoil may explain the reduction in angiographic restenosis and repeat revascularization after stenting. Neointimal hyperplasia, which results primarily from a growth response of the smooth muscle cells, is maximal at 1 to 4 weeks after the initial injury. Neointimal formation involves different steps: activation, proliferation, and migration of smooth muscle cells, as well as the production of extracellular matrix. De novo lesions are usually hypocellular, whereas restenotic lesions are typically hyperplastic.

Arterial remodeling plays an important role in restenosis. The changes in vessel size may be bidirectional: some lesions show an increase (enlargement) whereas others show a decrease (constriction) in vessel size. Stenting virtually eliminates late vascular remodeling.

In the hours following experimental angioplasty, endothelial cells rapidly enter the replication cycle to restore endothelial continuity. Endothelial regeneration starts from the leading edge of the denuded area and from the ostia of collateral and/or branch arteries (*Circulation* 1994;89:2816–2821), (*Circulation* 1993;88:I654), (*Lab Invest* 1978;39:141–150), (*Cardiovasc Res* 1996;31:835–846).

5.   Of the following statements regarding arterial remodeling after angioplasty, all are TRUE, **EXCEPT:**

    a. Restenosis after angioplasty is a balance between intimal formation and arterial remodeling.
    b. Arterial remodeling is described in de novo atherosclerosis as well as post angioplasty.
    c. Arterial remodeling is defined as constriction or "shrinkage" of the vessel with loss in coronary diameter after coronary intervention.
    d. Stents basically eliminate arterial remodeling.

ANSWER: c

Postangioplasty restenosis was initially attributed only to neointimal formation. Intravascular ultrasound (IVUS) studies have shown that several other possible responses to balloon injury may occur beside intimal formation: constriction as well as compensatory enlargement (*J Am Coll Cardiol* 1995;25:516–520). Arterial remodeling is well described in de novo atherosclerosis and after angioplasty. Animal studies have demonstrated compensatory arterial enlargement after angioplasty, limiting the effect of intimal formation on lumen narrowing; restenotic arteries had less arterial enlargement than nonrestenotic arteries. Compensatory enlargement and chronic constriction may represent two ends of the spectrum of arterial remodeling in response to angioplasty. Stents eliminate any component of arterial remodeling, either enlargement or constriction, and therefore reduce restenosis.

6. Of the following statements regarding late lumen loss, all are TRUE, **EXCEPT:**

   a. It represents the difference between the lumen diameter after the intervention and at 6 months' follow-up.
   b. It reflects the net effects of intimal hyperplasia (IH), elastic recoil, and vascular remodeling.
   c. Late loss averages 0.5 mm for PTCA and 0.9 mm for stents.
   d. The relationship between acute gain and late loss is constant among devices.

ANSWER: d

J Am Coll Cardiol 1993;2115–2125.

7. Of the following statements regarding aorto-coronary saphenous vein graft (SVG) disease, all are TRUE, **EXCEPT:**

   a. During the first year up to 15% of grafts occlude, between 1 and 6 years the attrition rate is 1% to 2% per year, and between 6 and 10 years it is 4% per year.
   b. Between 3% and 12% of grafts occlude within the first month, usually due to thrombosis.
   c. IH is the major disease process between 1 month and 1 year.
   d. Atherosclerosis is the dominant process beyond the first year; this is rarely significant before the third year.
   e. Severity of native disease proximal to the anastomosis does not influence SVG disease.

ANSWER: e

Angiographic patency at 1 year is 90% for SVG anastomosed to arteries with proximal stenosis greater than 70%, but only 80% for SVG anastomosed to arteries with proximal stenosis less than 70% (*Ann Thorac Surg* 1979;28:176–183).

8.   Of the following statements regarding acute vessel closure post PTCA, all are TRUE, **EXCEPT:**

    a. Approximately half of these will occur immediately postballoon inflation, and they are successfully treated with stents in more than 90% of cases.
    b. Up to 10% of late acute closures may not develop electrocardiographic (ECG) changes, especially if the intervention was performed in the circumflex artery or if there were well developed collaterals.
    c. The incidence of acute closure is around 15% of all interventions.
    d. Risk factors associated with death after acute closure include female gender, large ischemic burden, left ventricular function <30%, and proximal RCA PTCA.

ANSWER: c

Reported incidence of acute vessel closure is 2% to 7%; the incidence continues to decrease with improved equipment and antiplatelet therapy (*Ann Intern Med* 1997;127:458–471).

9.   Of the following statements about vascular access complications, all are TRUE, **EXCEPT:**

    a. Surgical repair is required in 0.9% to 3.5% of all procedures.
    b. Risk factors include preprocedural thrombolytic therapy, anticoagulation with warfarin, long-term use of corticosteroids, peripheral vascular disease, and female gender.
    c. Ultrasonography-guided compression of a pseudoaneurysm is successful in only 50% of cases.
    d. Early sheath removal, smaller diameter arterial sheaths, mechanical, or pneumatic compression devices may reduce vascular complications.

ANSWER: c

Pseudoaneurysms are treated successfully with compression in more than 80% of cases (*J Am Coll Cardiol* 1992;20:610–615).

10.   Which one of the following is NOT a risk factors for contrast-induced nephropathy?

   a. Preexisting renal dysfunction
   b. Amount but not type of contrast agent
   c. Diabetes mellitus
   d. Second dose of contrast within 72 hours
   e. Concomitant therapy with nonsteroidal anti-inflammatory agents

ANSWER: c

If not associated with renal disease, diabetes mellitus is NOT a risk factor for contrast-induced nephropathy (*N Engl J Med* 1989;320:143–149).

A second dose of contrast within 72 hours increases the risk by 40%. The only therapy that is proven to prevent nephropathy is I.V. hydration starting 12 hours before and continuing for 12 hours after contrast administration.

11.   Of the following statements regarding cholesterol embolization, all are TRUE, **EXCEPT:**

   a. It is due to microembolism of cholesterol crystals and other atherosclerotic debris after catheter manipulation resulting in occlusion of distal medium sized arteries.
   b. Laboratory test results include eosinophilia, eosinophiluria, elevated sedimentation rate, and decreased complement levels.
   c. Cutaneous manifestations include livedo reticularis, gangrene, and acrocyanosis.
   d. Nervous system manifestations include transient ischemic attacks, amaurosis fugax, and cranial and ocular paralysis.
   e. The triad of leg/foot pain, livedo reticularis, and intact peripheral pulses is considered pathognomonic.

ANSWER: a

The small arteries and arterioles (100 to 300 μm in diameter) are the ones affected. Definite diagnosis requires biopsy in conjunction with the clinical findings described. Unfortunately, there is no cure and the mortality rate is high (*Clin Cardiol* 1995;18: 609–614).

12.   All of the following are predictors of restenosis after stent implantation, **EXCEPT:**

    a. Not using IVUS
    b. Diabetes mellitus
    c. Multiple stents
    d. Minimal lumen diameter immediately post stenting
    e. Aorto-ostial lesions

ANSWER: a

Despite multiple studies showing that up to 30% of patients with an optimal angiographic result do NOT satisfy optimal deployment by IVUS criteria, no adverse clinical effects had been demonstrated as a consequence (*J Am Coll Cardiol* 1997;29[suppl A]:60A).

Match the following:

13.   Restenosis

14.   Recoil

15.   Remodeling

16.   Compensatory enlargement

    a. Local variation in arterial dimensions within the first minutes of angioplasty.
    b. A change in arterial caliber after coronary interventions.
    c. Lumen stenosis delay as lesion area increases.
    d. Local vascular response to wound healing associated with inevitable injury of balloon angioplasty.

ANSWERS: 13-d, 14-a, 15-b, 16-c

Restenosis encompasses the combined biologic healing processes (proliferative-, thrombotic-, or remodeling-derived), resulting in a renarrowing of the lumen after a transcatheter procedure (*Am Heart J* 1993;126:1243–1267).

There are two ways to define restenosis: binary definition (eg, percent stenosis 50% at follow-up), and continuous definitions.

Elastic recoil is a local variation in arterial dimensions immediately after the angioplasty; it reflects the difference between the diameter of the maximally inflated balloon and the resulting arterial minimal lumen diameter. It represents the immediate loss in lumen diameter upon balloon deflation (*Am J Cardiol* 1992;69:584–591).

Remodeling is the overall deformation of the arterial wall following coronary intervention. The early part of this response is the elastic recoil. Later, geometric remodeling occurs as the artery shrinks, owing to collagen deposition and fibrosis (*Am J Cardiol* 1998;81[7A]:4E-6E).

Glagov et al (*N Engl J Med* 1987;316:1371–1375) reported that human coronary arteries enlarge in relation to plaque area and that functionally important lumen stenosis may be delayed until the lesion occupies 40% of the internal elastic lamina area (compensatory enlargement).

17.   Of the following statements regarding myocardial cell death, all are TRUE, **EXCEPT:**

   a. During myocardial ischemia, myocardial cell metabolism becomes anaerobic and, consequently, myocardial cell hydrogen (H^+) concentration increases.
   b. During myocardial ischemia, there is a decrease in intracellular calcium (Ca^{++}).
   c. During reperfusion, more Ca^{++} enters the cell.
   d. Inhibition of the sodium/hydrogen (Na^+/H^+) exchange system would theoretically prevent or limit cell death.

ANSWER: b

During myocardial ischemia, myocardial cell metabolism becomes anaerobic and, consequently, intracellular hydrogen concentration increases. Via the Na^+/H^+ exchange, the hydrogen is exchanged for the sodium; as a result, sodium accumulates in the cell, leading to an increase in Ca^{++} by way of the Na^+/Ca^{++} exchange. The increased concentration of Ca^{++} causes cellular death. When reperfusion occurs, more sodium and calcium ions enter the cell causing myofibril injury (*Cardiovasc Res* 1995;29:184–188).

An agent that would inhibit the Na^+/H^+ exchange, would prevent the calcium overload and eventually prevent cellular death. An

Na^+/H^+ exchange inhibitor is currently used in clinical trials in patients undergoing PTCA, coronary artery bypass graft (CABG), and in patients with unstable angina and MI (GUARDIAN study).

Match the following:

18.   Modest reduction in the coronary blood flow and reduction of myocardial energy metabolism in a steady state, which may last months.

19.   Normal or high coronary flow and normal or excessive myocardial energy metabolism, lasting hours or days.

20.   Severely reduced coronary blood flow and increasingly reduced myocardial energy metabolism, lasting minutes to hours.

21.   Multiple short attacks of reduced coronary flow followed by complete reperfusion.

     a. Preconditioning
     b. True ischemia
     c. Stunning
     d. Hibernation

ANSWERS: 18-d, 19-c, 20-b, 21-a

Hibernation is the result of chronic hypoperfusion of the myocardium.

Radionuclide imaging techniques, positron-emission tomography (PET) scan and stress echocardiography (ECHO) can detect whether myocardial dysfunction is due to hibernation. This myocardium is viable but not contractile or is poorly contractile. The reduced contractility in hibernating myocardium reduces metabolism demands and may be protective. The predominant presenting symptoms may be secondary to left ventricular dysfunction and can be reversed by coronary revascularization.

Stunning is the result of transient ischemia (eg, exercise-induced ischemia, coronary spasm). The severity of stunning is greater in subendocardial layers of the left ventricular wall. The transient Ca^{++} overload, excitation-contraction uncoupling, and generation of free radicals upon reperfusion are most probable mechanisms involved. The recovery of stunned myocardium can take days. Patients frequently present with unstable angina.

True ischemia is secondary to severely reduced blood flow, which results in a progressive reduction of myocardial energy metabolism and leads to myocardial necrosis if not corrected.

Preconditioning represents brief episodes of ischemia followed by complete reperfusion resulting in a reduction in the amount of necrosis. The suggested mechanism may be related to a shortening in the action potential, decreases Ca^{++} influx, resulting in an energy-sparing effect. From a clinical standpoint, patients with multiple episodes of angina admitted with acute MI have a lower in-hospital mortality rate, a lower creatine phosphokinase (CPK) peak, and a lower rate of ventricular arrhythmias (*J Am Coll Cardiol* 1995;26:319).

22. Of the following statements regarding the vascular response to stenting, all are TRUE, **EXCEPT:**

   a. Preventing thrombus formation will affect late events.
   b. There are 4 distinct phases of vascular repair after stent-induced injury.
   c. There is a linear relationship between the number of monocytes per artery and the extent of arterial intimal growth.
   d. Insertion of a stent limits elastic recoil but not remodeling.

ANSWER: a

The 4 distinct phases of vascular reaction to stent implantation are:

1. Platelet-rich thrombus formation at the areas of deep stent injury peaking at 3 to 4 days after stent deployment, and accounting for most early luminal loss. Studies have shown that thrombus can be almost entirely prevented with no effect on later events (*Circulation* 1997;9:I710; *Circulation* 1997;95:1549–1553).
2. Inflammation starts concomitantly with thrombus deposition. Surface-adherent monocytes (SAMs) are recruited at the injury site. Between days 3 and 7 the SAMs migrate into neointima as tissue-infiltrating monocytes (TIMs), and remain there. The number of SAMs is the most powerful determinant of the rate of proliferation within the developed lesion (*Arterioscler Thromb Vasc Biol* 1996;16:1312–1318).

3. Proliferation of smooth muscle cells and mono-cytes/macrophages peaks at 7 days post stent implantation and continues for weeks. There is a linear relationship between the number of monocytes per artery and the extent of intimal growth.
4. Remodeling: although insertion of the stent limits the early part of remodeling (elastic recoil), it does not limit the whole process of remodeling. Collagen deposition, destruction of elastin, and inflamation are parts of the arterial response to the pressure of the stent struts.

Match the following:

23.   NO

24.   Metalloproteinase

25.   Endothelin

    a. Increases the vulnerability of fibrous cap.
    b. Modulates coronary autoregulation.
    c. Plasma concentration is elevated in atherosclerosis, congestive heart failure (CHF) and acute MI.

ANSWER: 23-b, 24-a, 25-c

Endothelium plays an important role in coronary autoregulation through the generation of vasoactive and growth-regulatory substances.

Production of NO in response to hemodynamic and chemical stimuli is the primary mechanism by which endothelium regulates smooth muscle tone and proliferation (*Circ Res* 1995;76: 305–309). NO is a potent inhibitor of platelet aggregation and monocyte adhesion.

The integrity of the fibrous cap is maintained by extracellular matrix molecules. Endothelium, smooth muscle cells, and macrophages produce a group of enzymes called metalloproteinases, which are able to degrade matrix components. There is an increased metalloproteinase activity in the vulnerable shoulder region of the plaques, which may lead to weakening and rupture (*J Clin Invest* 1994;94:2493–2503).

Endothelins are peptides with potent vasoconstrictor activity. Endothelin-1 (the only endothelin produced by the endothelium) has a longer activity than NO (minutes or hours versus a few seconds). Agents that stimulate endothelin-1 production are: thrombin, angiotensin II, epinephrine, and vasopressin. The effect of endothelin is vasoconstriction. Endothelin is also produced by activated macrophages present in ruptured plaques responsible for acute coronary syndromes (Braunwald E. *Heart Disease: A Textbook of Cardiovascular Medicine.* Philadelphia: W.B. Saunders Co.; 1997: 1167–1168).

26.   The two factors that passivate platelets at the endothelial level are:

   a. Prostaglandin I-2 and NO
   b. Endothelium-derived relaxing factor and NO
   c. Prostaglandin I-2 and PGI_2

ANSWER: a

Endothelial cells have metabolic properties which allow preservation of blood fluidity under normal circumstances.

The two endothelium-derived factors that passivate platelets are PGI_2 (known as prostaglandin I-2) and NO (also known as endothelial-derived relaxing factor).

These inhibitors of platelet activation are labile molecules acting in proximity of the endothelium. PGI_2 stimulates platelet adenyl cyclase and NO stimulates platelet guanylyl cyclase, therefore raising intraplatelet levels of cAMP and cGMP, respectively. The cAMP and cGMP levels are elevated as well at the level of subendothelial smooth muscle cells, rendering to PGI_2 and NO the properties of potent vasorelaxants and mediators of vascular tone (*Cardiovascular Therapeutics: A Companion to Braunwald's Heart Disease.* Philadelphia: W.B. Saunders Co.; 1996:427).

Match the following:

27.   Activated partial thromboplastin time (aPTT)

28.   Prothrombin time (PT)

29.   Vitamin K

30.   Protein C, Protein S

    a. Intrinsic pathway
    b. Anticoagulants
    c. Extrinsic pathway
    d. Platelet membrane glycoproteins
    e. g-Carboxylation of glutamic acid residues

ANSWERS: 27-a, 28-c, 29-e, 30-b

The intrinsic pathway begins with the activation of factor XII and subsequently factor XI by thrombin and the presence of negatively charged surfaces. Factor XIa then activates factor IX, which, in complex with factor VIIa (activated by thrombin), activate factor X.

The extrinsic pathway, tissue factor binds to factor VII. They then activate factors IX and X and thereafter the common pathway is activated. Factor Xa forms a complex with factor Va (again activated by thrombin), and calcium will cleave prothrombin, creating thrombin. This will generate fibrin from fibrinogen.

The regulation of the coagulation cascade is accomplished with antithrombin III (AT III), which binds thrombin and is greatly accelerated by heparin. Protein C and its cofactor, protein S (both are also vitamin K-dependent), are activated by thrombin and inactivate factors VIII and V.

Tissue factor inhibitor binds to factor Xa, and this complex in turn binds to the tissue factor-factor VIII complex, thus inactivating the extrinsic pathway. However, the mechanism responsible for maintaining this balance is not known.

The vitamin K-dependent proteins undergo g-carboxylation of 10 to 12 specific glutamic acid residues before they are secreted from the hepatocyte; these are located on the propeptide of prothrombin, protein C, protein S, and factors IX, X, and VII . The vitamin K-dependent carboxylase, in the presence of reduced vitamin K, fixes carbon dioxide to form the new carboxyl group on the glutamic acid, and simultaneously converts the vitamin K to vitamin K epoxide. This is salvaged by conversion to vitamin K by the epoxide reductase, which is sensitive to warfarin (*N Engl J Med* 1992;326:800–806).

Match the following:

31.   Unstable angina

32.   Non Q wave MI

33.   Transmural MI

    a.   White thrombus
    b.   Red thrombus

ANSWERS: 31-a, 32-a, 33-b

The thrombi of patients with unstable angina and non Q wave MI appear grayish white on angioscopy. The white thrombus is composed of platelets and fibrin. This type of thrombus is more resistant to thrombolytic therapy.

The red thrombus is seen in patients with acute transmural MI, and is composed of erythrocytes, fibrin, platelets, and leukocytes. This thrombus responds favorably to thrombolytic therapy (Braunwald E. *Heart Disease. A Textbook of Cardiovascular Medicine.* 5th ed. Philadelphia: W.B. Saunders Co., 1997:1187).

34.   Of the following statements regarding the comparison between SVGs and internal mammary artery (IMA) conduits, all are TRUE, **EXCEPT:**

    a.   Accelerated atherosclerosis appears commonly in SVGs but is uncommon in IMA conduits.
    b.   The internal elastic lamina of IMA is uniform and the media has metabolic supply from the lumen and from vasa vasorum.
    c.   IMA diameter more frequently matches the bypassed artery diameter.
    d.   The vasodilatatory response is more pronounced in SVGs.

ANSWER: d

The endothelium of arterial conduits produces more PGI_2 than SVGs, and the endothelium-dependent relaxation is more significant in arterial conduits (*Am Heart J* 1991;122:1192). It has to be mentioned, though, that the vein conduits preserve their capacity to vasodilate when nitroglycerin is given intravasculary (*Circulation* 1997;96[10]:3785–3786).

The 10 to 12 years' follow-up shows a patency rate of greater than 90% for IMA grafts and only 40% to 60% for vein grafts (*Curr Probl Surg* 1992;29:756).

35.   During rotational atherectomy, platelet aggregation is:

    a. Not affected
    b. Dependent on burr diameter
    c. Dependent on burr speed

ANSWER: c

Platelet aggregability is increased at higher speeds (*J Am Coll Cardiol* 1997;27:186A).

The problem with using lower speeds (75,000 rpm) is that the particles generated are larger (*Circulation* 1988;72:II83). Currently, a clinical registry is in course to establish whether lower speeds are associated with less untoward effects.

36.   Microcavitation is associated with which one of the following atherectomy devices?

    a. Rotablation
    b. Transluminal extraction catheter (TEC)
    c. Excimer laser
    d. Endoluminal radiation using iridium

ANSWER: a

The critical speed for dissolving gas-forming bubbles (microcavitation) in blood is 14.7 m/s. This speed is reached by rotablation device.

Experiments in vitro showed that the mean bubble size resulting from high-speed rotational atherectomy in fresh whole blood is 90±33 μm. These bubbles collapse in less than 10 seconds; to date, there is no evidence that these cavitation bubbles may have clinical implications (*Cathet Cardiovasc Diagn* 1992;26:98–109).

37.   Intimal dissection after balloon angioplasty is associated with increased risk of:

   a. Restenosis
   b. Restenosis and acute closure
   c. Acute closure
   d. None of the above

ANSWER: c

The presence of dissection after PTCA does not correlate with increased rate of restenosis (*J Am Coll Cardiol* 1995;25:139A; *J Am Coll Cardiol* 1995;25:345A).

On the other hand, intimal dissection is the most powerful predictor of acute closure, especially the presence of dissections of type C through F (*Circulation* 1988;77:372–379).

The overwhelming majority of dissections disappear in 3 to 6 months after the procedure.

38.   Of the following statements regarding reperfusion therapy for acute MI, all are TRUE, **EXCEPT:**

   a. Thrombolytic therapy is associated with recurrent ischemia in 15% to 30% of cases.
   b. PTCA is associated with better immediate patency rates.
   c. PTCA offers better survival in high-risk patients.
   d. Patients who received thrombolytic therapy should undergo angiography before discharge to define coronary anatomy and need for revascularization.

ANSWER: d

Present data do not support the routine use of angiography for asymptomatic patients who have received thrombolytics, unless they develop post-MI angina, have a positive stress test, or have a history of prior MI. In these situations revascularization is appropriate.

Indeed, thrombolytic therapy is associated with 15% to 30% recurrent ischemia.

Primary PTCA offers better patency rates (>95%) than primary thrombolytic therapy.

High-risk patients have better survival rates when treated with primary PTCA (*N Engl J Med* 1993;328:673–679).

Chapter 3

Pharmacotherapy

QUESTIONS

1. What is the dosage for abciximab (ReoPro; Centocor, Malvern, PA)?

    a. 0.25 mg/kg I.V. bolus followed by a continuous I.V. infusion of 0.125 μg/kg/min (to a maximum of 10 mg/min) for 12 hours.

    b. 25 mg/kg I.V. bolus followed by a continuous I.V. infusion of 0.125 mg/kg/min for 12 hours.

    c. 25 mg bolus for patients weighing <75 kg and 50 mg bolus for patients weighing more than 75 kg, followed by 12 hours of continuous I.V. infusion of 0.125 mg/kg/min.

2. What is the target activated clotting time (ACT) for patients receiving abciximab?

    a. 150 to 200 seconds
    b. 200 to 300 seconds
    c. 300 to 350 seconds
    d. More than 350 seconds, if adjunctive heparin is not used

3. What are the usual glycoprotein IIb/IIIa (Gp IIb/IIIa) receptor blockade and percent platelet aggregation relative to baseline in patients treated with abciximab?

    a. 80% and 20%, respectively
    b. 50% and 50%, respectively
    c. 20% and 80%, respectively

4. Which of the following is a contraindication for the use of abciximab?

    a. History of cerebrovascular accident (CVA) within 2 years.
    b. Thrombocytopenia (<100,000).
    c. Vasculitis.
    d. Use of dextran.
    e. All of the above.

5.   What is the initial half-life of abciximab?

    a. 10 minutes
    b. 1 hour
    c. 4 hours
    d. 6 hours

6.   You are performing an angioplasty, the patient had received abciximab (ReoPro), and there is a need for emergent coronary bypass surgery. Current available data support stopping ReoPro and:

    a. Sending the patient to the operating room (OR) immediately.
    b. Trying to stabilize the patient and waiting 24 to 48 hours before the surgery.
    c. Transfusing platelets and send the patient to the OR.
    d. Checking platelet function.

7.   A 68-year-old social worker is admitted to the critical care unit (CCU) after having had 3 episodes of resting angina in the last 48 hours. He has a vague history of hypertension and he is a heavy smoker. He weighs 90 kg, and is in no apparent distress. He states that his chest feels "heavy." His BP is 150/100 mm Hg and his HR is 71 bpm. Physical examination is unremarkable except for an S4 at the apex and scattered crackles bilaterally. Chest x-ray shows a normal heart size and no congestion. ECG shows normal sinus rhythm and ST-T depression in leads II, III, and aVF while he complains of chest pain. You start him on β-blockers, aspirin, heparin I.V., to keep the PTT between 60 and 80, and nitroglycerin drip. He is symptom-free for a few hours but at 4:00 PM the CCU nurse notifies you that the patient has had another episode of chest pain, which was relieved after two tablets of sublingual nitroglycerin and 4 mg of morphine sulphate I.V. He is now asleep; BP is 120/70 mm Hg, HR is 55 bpm, and there are no ECG changes. The first two sets of enzymes are negative and the troponin is positive.

What would you do next?

    a. You give him 75 mg tissue plasminogen activator (tPA) over 90 minutes and schedule him for angiography/possible PTCA at 10:00 AM the next day.

   b. You give him 0.8 mg/kg tPA over 90 minutes and schedule him for coronary angiography only after failure of the initial treatment.

   c. You perform an emergent angiography and find out that he has a 90% stenosis in proximal RCA (dominant system) associated with large thrombus burden; you give him 150,000 U of urokinase I.C. and proceed with PTCA, followed by an additional 250,00 U of urokinase I.C.

   d. You give him a bolus (0.25 mg/kg) followed by an infusion (10 µg/min) of abciximab and schedule him for angiography/angioplasty the next morning.

8.   Management of coronary spasm in the setting of PTCA includes all of the following, **EXCEPT:**

   a. Repeat balloon dilatation at low-pressure inflation.
   b. Anticholinergic therapy.
   c. Emergency bypass surgery.
   d. The use of I.C. nitrates for distal microvascular spasm.

9.   Regarding aspirin for SVG disease:

   a. It improves patency at 1 year post bypass; its effect, however, is markedly dependent on grafted native vessel diameter, such that vessels larger than 2 mm may not benefit from aspirin.
   b. It is effective if commenced no later than 1 day after the surgery (ineffective after the third day).
   c. It has not been proven to improve patency rates between 1 and 3 years after surgery.
   d. Ticlopidine is NOT an adequate alternative, due to lack of studies in this group of patients.

10.   Of the following statements regarding the role of probucol in restenosis, all are TRUE, **EXCEPT:**

   a. It protects LDL from oxidation.
   b. It is incorporated in LDL.
   c. Pretreatment is essential.
   d. The effect is dose-dependent.
   e. It does not affect high-density lipoprotein (HDL).

11.   Of the following statements regarding acute severe thrombocytopenia due to abciximab, all are TRUE, **EXCEPT:**

    a.   It is defined as a platelet count <100,000/μL within 24
       hours of treatment.
    b.   Platelet transfusions should be given.
    c.   Differential diagnosis includes type II heparin-induced
       thrombocytopenia (HIT).
    d.   If it develops, abciximab should be discontinued.

12.   A 58-year-old man is referred to you for an angioplasty of
a 95% stenosis in a 2.8 mm diameter left circumflex coronary
artery (LCX). An angioplasty is successfully performed, with a less
than 20% residual stenosis and a type B dissection. You decide
that starting the patient on enoxaparin 40 mg/day will:

    a.   Decrease the risk of restenosis.
    b.   Decrease the risk of recurrent angina.
    c.   Increase the performance in exercise stress test at 24
       weeks.
    d.   Not affect the outcome in any way.

13.   Of the following statements regarding eptifibatide (Integrilin; COR Therapeutics, South San Francisco, CA) treatment, all
are TRUE, **EXCEPT:**

    a.   It is used concomitantly with heparin and aspirin.
    b.   It decreases the rate of death and MI in patients with
       acute coronary syndromes.
    c.   During the infusion the aPTT should be maintained be-
       tween 50 and 70 seconds.
    d.   It is cleared equally by renal and nonrenal mecha-
       nisms.
    e.   Age is not a contraindication to treatment.

14.   Heparin is used routinely during angioplasty to prevent
abrupt vessel closure. All of the following are true properties of
heparin, **EXCEPT:**

    a.   Heparin is able to bind to AT III.
    b.   Nonanticoagulant fractions are as effective as the anti-

coagulant fractions in prevention of neointimal proliferation.

c. The antiproliferative effect is dose-dependent and
greater for low molecular weight heparin (LMWH).

d. The antiproliferative action is related to incorporation
into the cell membrane.

15.   The revised labeling for the use of Glucophage in patients
with type II diabetes requiring studies using iodinated contrast
materials contains all of the following, **EXCEPT:**

a. Special recommendations pertain only to those cases
that require intravascular administration.

b. Current Glucophage treatment is a contraindication to
using contrast dye.

c. Glucophage should be withheld for 48 hours after the
procedure.

d. Glucophage should be stopped at the time of the procedure.

16.   Of the following statements regarding the use of ticlopidine, all are TRUE, **EXCEPT:**

a. It has been associated with thrombotic thrombocytopenic purpura (TTP), a rare complication, with a
high mortality rate, that is difficult to predict.

b. The incidence of neutropenia is 2.4%; it is usually reversible when the drug is stopped.

c. It increases serum cholesterol by approximately 8% to
10%.

d. It has a delayed onset of action, making it inappropriate for acute management.

17.   Of the following statements regarding aspirin, all are
TRUE, **EXCEPT:**

a. It selectively acetylates the hydroxyl group of a serine
residue of the platelet prostaglandin G/H synthase 1
(cyclooxygenase), resulting in decrease conversion of
arachidonate to ultimately thromboxane A2.

b. The dose required to almost completely suppress the

biosynthesis of thromboxane A2 is 100 mg; this is a cumulative effect, thus lower daily dosages are needed thereafter (usually 30 to 50 mg).

c. Gastrointestinal bleeding and probably intracranial bleeding are side effects that are dose-dependent.

d. It decreases the incidence of acute coronary occlusion after angioplasty by 50% when given before the procedure.

e. Aspirin may enhance some of the beneficial effects of angiotensin-converting inhibitors in patients with ischemic cardiomyopathy and severe congestive heart failure.

18.   Which one of the following patients should not receive protamine?

a. A 50-year-old woman with myasthenia gravis.

b. A 62-year-old woman with end-stage renal disease, on hemodialysis.

c. A 65-year-old patient whose diabetes is well controlled with neutral protamine Hagedorn (NPH) insulin.

d. 40-year-old man who has a documented intracranial atrioventricular (AV) malformation.

19.   A 55-year-old woman is admitted with unstable angina. She is treated with β-blockers, aspirin, I.V. nitroglycerin, and heparin. Despite maximum medical treatment, she continues to have brief episodes of resting angina; therefore she is referred for coronary angiography, which reveals a 90% stenosis of the mid left anterior descending (LAD) coronary artery. She undergoes percutaneous revascularization and a stent is placed at the site of the stenosis. An excellent result is obtained, with 0% residual stenosis. The patient is discharged home in 48 hours, on β-blockers, aspirin 325 mg by mouth (P.O.), every day (QD), and ticlopidine 250 mg P.O., QD for 2 weeks only. You see her in your office at 2 weeks after her angioplasty; she is symptom-free and plans to return to work next week. Eight days after her last visit, you receive a telephone call from her family and learn that she was admitted emergently to the hospital 2 hours ago with confusion, fever, and a skin rash. You order blood work stat. Which one of the following tests is more likely to be normal?

    a. Hemoglobin
    b. Creatinine
    c. Lactic dehydrogenase (LDH)
    d. PT/PTT

20.   Regarding the syndrome that the patient discussed above developed, which one of the following statements is TRUE?

    a. Hemolytic anemia, thrombocytopenia, neurological symptoms, fever, and renal dysfunction represent the pentad of symptoms characterizing the syndrome.
    b. This is an immune process causing platelet destruction.
    c. Closer monitoring of count cell/chemistry would have ensued earlier diagnosis.
    d. Early biopsy of the skin, muscle, and gingiva would have helped in the diagnosis.

Match the following:

21.   Heparin

22.   Hirudin

23.   Argatroban

24.   Integrilin

25.   Tirofiban

    a. Direct inhibitor of thrombin
    b. Indirect inhibitor of thrombin
    c. Fibrinogen receptor antagonist

26.   The term *passivation* refers to:

    a. Switching from a regular balloon to a perfusion balloon in patients with low tolerance for pain, allowing longer balloon inflations.
    b. Performing a percutaneous revascularization proce-

dure on a patient under general anesthesia, mostly in patients who cannot lie flat because of CHF.
c. The change in an arterial surface from one that supports platelet deposition to one that does not.
d. A property of a material to be deformed continuously and permanently without rupture (eg, stents).

27.   Of the following statements regarding nitrate therapy, all are TRUE, **EXCEPT:**

a. They all go extensive first-pass hepatic metabolism when given orally, except the mononitrates.
b. They ultimately act through liberation of NO by the endothelium.
c. I.C. nitroglycerin is the drug of choice for "no reflow" phenomena.
d. Tolerance develops if no daily nitrate-free period is given.

28.   All of the following statements regarding the synthetic nonpeptide inhibitors of GpIIb/IIIa receptor are TRUE, **EXCEPT:**

a. They are reversible antagonists, with a shorter effect than monoclonal antibodies.
b. They are not immunogenic.
c. They can be given orally.
d. They have not yet been tested in humans.

29.   Of the following statements regarding thrombocytopenia in a patient who underwent a coronary artery intervention, all are TRUE, **EXCEPT:**

a. The rate of thrombocytopenia induced by abciximab (chimeric 7E3 Fab) second administration is 6% to 7%.
b. The time frame of HIT is different from that of thrombocytopenia induced by readministration of abciximab.
c. The medical treatment is the same for HIT and abciximab-induced thrombocytopenia.
d. The platelet count of patients treated with abciximab should be drawn in 3 separate tubes (on citrate, edetic acid [EDTA], and heparin).

30.   The use of thrombolytic therapy in the setting of angioplasty performed for unstable angina is:

   a. Strongly indicated because of the presence of thrombus,
      frequently present in unstable coronary syndromes.
   b. Indicated only in cases in which dissection and throm-
      bus are evident on angiography.
   c. Not indicated because, in association with heparin, the
      risk of bleeding increases prohibitively.
   d. Not generally indicated because of poorer outcome.

Match the following:

31.   tPA

32.   Streptokinase

33.   Urokinase

34.   Reteplase

   a. Binds to plasminogen and then activates it
   b. Cleaves a peptide bond of plasminogen, activating it

35.   Of the following medical therapies, which one is correct
for the treatment of contrast-dye–related anaphylactic shock?

   a. Draw 1 mL of 1:1000 epinephrine, and dilute it to a
      total volume of 10 mL (10 µg/mL). Then adminis-
      ter it I.V., 1 mL every (Q) 1 minute, until BP is re-
      stored.
   b. Administer boluses of 10 µg of epinephrine Q 1 minute
      until the desired BP is obtained, and continue with an
      I.V. infusion of 1 to 4 µg/min to maintain the BP at the
      desired level.
   c. Administer 0.3 cc of 1:1000 solution subcutaneously
      (S.Q.) Q 15 minutes up to 1 mL.
   d. Rapid administration of 1 mg I.V. of epinephrine will
      restore the BP in 90% of cases.

36.   Of the following statements regarding adjunctive therapy for stents, all are FALSE, **EXCEPT:**

a. The treatment with aspirin and ticlopidine has comparable impact on stent thrombosis to that with aspirin and warfarin, but has less bleeding complications.
b. Warfarin therapy should be used as an adjunctive medication only in cases of suboptimal stent deployment.
c. Prophylactic antibiotic therapy should be used according to the same criteria employed for valvular diseases.
d. If a patient is allergic/intolerant to ticlopidine, clopidogrel can be used instead.

Match the following:

37.   Ticlopidine

38.   Aspirin

39.   Clopidogrel

40.   Tirofiban

a. Inhibits thromboxane formation.
b. Inhibits adenosine diphosphate- (ADP) mediated activation of the GpIIb/IIIa complex.
c. Nonprotein reversible antagonist of the platelet GpIIb/IIIa receptor.

41.   Which of the following is recommended for the use of heparin after PTCA?

a. Discontinue immediately.
b. Continue at full strength for an additional 6 to 12 hours.
c. Continue at full strength for 24 hours, during sheath removal use half-strength.

42.   Patients with history of HIT who are to undergo angioplasty may receive instead all of the following, **EXCEPT:**

a. LMWH
b. Hirudin
c. Bivalirudin (Hirulog)
d. Abciximab

43. Which one of the following measures reduces restenosis after PTCA in small coronary arteries (diameter <2.5 mm)?

a. High-dose multivitamins
b. Probucol
c. High-dose multivitamins combined with probucol
d. Stenting

44. Of the following statements regarding coronary vasodilatation, all are TRUE, **EXCEPT:**

a. Nitroglycerin I.C. has a more predictive response than sublingual (S.L.) or I.V. nitroglycerin.
b. Ionic contrast agents may induce vasodilatation up to 20%.
c. Nonionic contrast agents produce more vasodilatation than ionic agents.
d. The effect of I.C. nitroglycerin peaks at 1 minute.

45. Which one of the following statements is TRUE regarding the aspirin/ticlopidine (A/T) combination compared to aspirin/warfarin (A/W) combination?

a. A/T results in less bleeding complications but higher in-stent acute thrombosis.
b. A/T results in less bleeding complications and less in-stent thrombosis.
c. A/T combination results in the same clinical outcome provided the warfarin is given to maintain an international normalized ratio (INR) above 3.0.
d. There are no data to support the benefit of one therapy over the other.

46. Of the following statements regarding aspirin allergy, all are TRUE, **EXCEPT:**

a. Patients with asthma and rhino-sinusitis may develop aspirin sensitivity.
b. Desensitization involves administering progressively higher doses of aspirin at specific time intervals.
c. Patients with aspirin-induced angio-edema, urticaria, or anaphylaxis should not undergo desensitization.
d. A cutaneous reaction to aspirin puts the patient at risk for anaphylaxis upon readministration of the drug.
e. A patient who underwent successful desensitization but interrupted his or her aspirin for 3 days during a hiking trip requires a new desensitization attempt.

ANSWERS

1. What is the dosage for abciximab (ReoPro; Centocor, Malvern, PA)?

   a. 0.25 mg/kg I.V. bolus followed by a continuous I.V. infusion of 0.125 µg/kg/min (to a maximum of 10 mg/min) for 12 hours.
   b. 25 mg/kg I.V. bolus followed by a continuous I.V. infusion of 0.125 mg/kg/min for 12 hours.
   c. 25 mg bolus for patients weighing <75 kg and 50 mg bolus for patients weighing more than 75 kg, followed by 12 hours of continuous I.V. infusion of 0.125 mg/kg/min.

ANSWER: a

In the EPIC and EPILOG trials, the dose of abciximab used was 0.25 mg/kg I.V. bolus followed by 12 hours' infusion of 0.125 µg/kg/min.

2. What is the target activated clotting time (ACT) for patients receiving abciximab?

   a. 150 to 200 seconds
   b. 200 to 300 seconds
   c. 300 to 350 seconds
   d. More than 350 seconds, if adjunctive heparin is not used

ANSWER: b

The target ACT for patients receiving abciximab is 200 to 300 seconds. The following regimen is used:

ACT less than 150 seconds: heparin bolus of 70 U/kg (EPILOG; *N Engl J Med* 1997;336:1689–1696).

ACT 150 to 199 seconds: 50 U/kg heparin.

ACT greater than 200 seconds: **No** heparin.

3. What are the usual glycoprotein IIb/IIIa (Gp IIb/IIIa) receptor blockade and percent platelet aggregation relative to baseline in patients treated with abciximab?

   a. 80% and 20%, respectively
   b. 50% and 50%, respectively
   c. 20% and 80%, respectively

ANSWER: a

Greater than 80% receptor blockade and less than 20% platelet function (measured by ex vivo platelet aggregation in response to ADP and bleeding time >30 minutes).

4.   Which of the following is a contraindication for the use of abciximab?

    a. History of cerebrovascular accident (CVA) within 2 years.
    b. Thrombocytopenia (<100,000).
    c. Vasculitis.
    d. Use of dextran.
    e. All of the above.

ANSWER: e

The contraindications for the use of abciximab are as follows:

- Active internal bleeding.
- History of CVA within 2 years.
- Thrombocytopenia (<100,000/mL)
- Recent surgery or trauma (within 6 weeks).
- Known intracranial neoplasm, AV malformation or aneurism.
- Vasculitis.
- Use of Dextran.

5.   What is the initial half-life of abciximab?

    a. 10 minutes
    b. 1 hour
    c. 4 hours
    d. 6 hours

ANSWER: a

The initial half-life of 10 minutes is followed by a second-phase half-life of 30 minutes. Platelet function recovers over the course of 48 hours after the termination of the infusion.

6.   You are performing an angioplasty, the patient had received abciximab (ReoPro), and there is a need for emergent coronary bypass surgery. Current available data support stopping ReoPro and:

a. Sending the patient to the operating room (OR) immediately.
b. Trying to stabilize the patient and waiting 24 to 48 hours before the surgery.
c. Transfusing platelets and send the patient to the OR.
d. Checking platelet function.

ANSWER: a

Although the data are limited, abciximab was not associated with excess major bleeding in patients who underwent CABG surgery (the range among all treatment arms was 3% to 5% in the EPIC trial, and 1% to 2% in the CAPTURE and EPILOG trials). However, some patients received platelet transfusions prior to surgery. Since platelet transfusions are also associated with risk, generally transfusions are given as clinically indicated to control bleeding, but not as a preventive measure.

7.   A 68-year-old social worker is admitted to the critical care unit (CCU) after having had 3 episodes of resting angina in the last 48 hours. He has a vague history of hypertension and he is a heavy smoker. He weighs 90 kg, and is in no apparent distress. He states that his chest feels "heavy." His BP is 150/100 mm Hg and his HR is 71 bpm. Physical examination is unremarkable except for an S4 at the apex and scattered crackles bilaterally. Chest x-ray shows a normal heart size and no congestion. ECG shows normal sinus rhythm and ST-T depression in leads II, III, and aVF while he complains of chest pain. You start him on β-blockers, aspirin, heparin I.V., to keep the PTT between 60 and 80, and nitroglycerin drip. He is symptom-free for a few hours but at 4:00 PM the CCU nurse notifies you that the patient has had another episode of chest pain, which was relieved after two tablets of sublingual nitroglycerin and 4 mg of morphine sulphate I.V. He is now asleep; BP is 120/70 mm Hg, HR is 55 bpm, and there are no ECG changes. The first two sets of enzymes are negative and the troponin is positive.

What would you do next?

a. You give him 75 mg tissue plasminogen activator (tPA) over 90 minutes and schedule him for angiography/possible PTCA at 10:00 AM the next day.
b. You give him 0.8 mg/kg tPA over 90 minutes and schedule him for coronary angiography only after failure of the initial treatment.
c. You perform an emergent angiography and find out that he has a 90% stenosis in proximal RCA (dominant system) associated with large thrombus burden; you give him 150,000 U of urokinase I.C. and proceed with PTCA, followed by an additional 250,00 U of urokinase I.C.
d. You give him a bolus (0.25 mg/kg) followed by an infusion (10 μg/min) of abciximab and schedule him for angiography/angioplasty the next morning.

ANSWER: d

The CAPTURE (Chimeric 7E3 Anti-Platelet Therapy in Unstable angina Refractory to standard treatment) trial was prematurely stopped because of the positive findings at an interim analysis (*Circulation* 1996;93:637). This international, multicenter trial included patients with unstable angina who were scheduled for PTCA. The patients were treated with aspirin, I.V. heparin, and a bolus (0.25 mg/kg) followed by an infusion (10 μg/min) of abciximab, which was initiated 18 to 24 hours before PTCA and continued for 1 hour after the procedure. The interim analysis in 1050 patients showed a significant reduction (10.8% versus 16.4%; $P<0.01$) in composite clinical endpoints of MI, need for urgent revascularization, and mortality at 30 days after PTCA. At 6 months the beneficial effect was less evident.

Thrombolytic therapy is not recommended unless the ECG demonstrates ST segment elevation or left bundle branch block ([LBBB] presumed to be new). The TIMI-IIIB trial (*Circulation* 1994;89:1545–1556) randomized 1473 patients with unstable angina to tPA plus heparin versus heparin for the initial treatment. Fatal and nonfatal MI at 42 days occurred more frequently in tPA-treated patients than in controls (7.4% versus 4.9%).

In the TAUSA trial (*Circulation* 1994;90:69–77), 469 patients with resting angina were randomized to placebo or I.C. urokinase. Although the angiographic endpoint of thrombus showed a trend toward reduction with urokinase, the incidence of abrupt vessel closure was increased with the adjunctive use of urokinase (10.2% versus 4.3%; $P<0.02$). There was also an increase in occurrence of recurrent ischemia, MI, or emergency CABG (12.9% versus 6.3%; $P<0.02$).

8.   Management of coronary spasm in the setting of PTCA includes all of the following, **EXCEPT:**

   a.   Repeat balloon dilatation at low-pressure inflation.
   b.   Anticholinergic therapy.
   c.   Emergency bypass surgery.
   d.   The use of I.C. nitrates for distal microvascular spasm.

ANSWER: d

In contrast to epicardial spasm, spasm of the distal microvascular bed rarely responds to nitrates. I.C. administration of verapamil (100 to 200 μg; total dose up to 1.0 to 1.5 mg) or diltiazem (0.5 to 2.5 mg bolus; total dose up to 5 to 10 mg) has been shown to reverse the distal microvascular spasm (*Circulation* 1994;89: 2514–2518).

If intralesional spasm persists despite intracoronary nitrates, a prolonged (2 to 5 minutes) low-pressure (1 to 4 atm) inflation using a balloon matched to the reference vessel is frequently successful in relieving the spasm.

Acetylcholine may induce paradoxical vasoconstriction in de-endothelialized arteries, probably due to local loss of endothelial-derived relaxing factor. In this case, spasm is accompanied by signs of vagal hypertony and can be treated with atropine 0.5 mg I.V. every 5 minutes to a total of 2.0 mg.

In the face of ongoing ischemia secondary to refractory spasm of a vessel suitable for grafting, emergency bypass should be considered if there is a large area of jeopardized myocardium.

9.   Regarding aspirin for SVG disease:

   a. It improves patency at 1 year post bypass; its effect, however, is markedly dependent on grafted native vessel diameter, such that vessels larger than 2 mm may not benefit from aspirin.
   b. It is effective if commenced no later than 1 day after the surgery (ineffective after the third day).
   c. It has not been proven to improve patency rates between 1 and 3 years after surgery.
   d. Ticlopidine is NOT an adequate alternative, due to lack of studies in this group of patients.

ANSWER: d

Two placebo-controlled trials demonstrated the effectiveness of ticlopidine (500 mg/day started from the second postoperative day) (*J Thorac Cardiovasc Surg* 1987;94:773–783). However, there are no data comparing it with aspirin or, even further, combining the two drugs.

10.   Of the following statements regarding the role of probucol in restenosis, all are TRUE, **EXCEPT:**

   a. It protects LDL from oxidation.
   b. It is incorporated in LDL.

    c. Pretreatment is essential.
    d. The effect is dose-dependent.
    e. It does not affect high-density lipoprotein (HDL).

ANSWER: e

Probucol lowers the levels of LDL and protects LDL from oxidation and the cells from toxic effects of oxidized lipoprotein. Whereas other supposed antioxidants are hydrosoluble (vitamin C, heparin), probucol and α-tocopherol are liposoluble (therefore incorporated in the LDL particle).

The process needs time (pretreatment is essential!). The higher the dose, the stronger the effect.

For every 1% decrease in LDL, there is a 3% decrease in HDL.

11.   Of the following statements regarding acute severe thrombocytopenia due to abciximab, all are TRUE, **EXCEPT:**

    a. It is defined as a platelet count $<100,000/\mu L$ within 24 hours of treatment.
    b. Platelet transfusions should be given.
    c. Differential diagnosis includes type II heparin-induced thrombocytopenia (HIT).
    d. If it develops, abciximab should be discontinued.

ANSWER: b

Only patients who are actively bleeding need the transfusion (usually 6 units of random-donor or 1 unit single-donor platelet pheresis if available) at this level. Otherwise the threshold for prophylactic transfusion is $20,000/\mu L$ (*Blood* 1993;81: 1411–1413), although some would consider transfusion at $50,000/\mu L$.

A platelet count check is recommended between 2 to 4 hours after the abciximab bolus; additional measures include strict bed rest, no intramuscular injections, stool softeners, and platelet counts every 12 hours. PT, aPTT, plasma fibrinogen level, D-dimer titre, and heparin-dependent antibody should also be performed.

The mechanism of thrombocytopenia is unknown (*Circulation* 1997;95:809–813).

12.   A 58-year-old man is referred to you for an angioplasty of a 95% stenosis in a 2.8 mm diameter left circumflex coronary artery (LCX). An angioplasty is successfully performed, with a less than 20% residual stenosis and a type B dissection. You decide that starting the patient on enoxaparin 40 mg/day will:

    a. Decrease the risk of restenosis.
    b. Decrease the risk of recurrent angina.
    c. Increase the performance in exercise stress test at 24 weeks.
    d. Not affect the outcome in any way.

ANSWER: d

The Enoxaparin Restenosis Trial (*Circulation* 1994;90:908–914) showed that enoxaparin given S.Q. for 24 days after PTCA does not reduce the occurrence of restenosis (51% placebo versus 52% enoxaparin group) or the rate of adverse clinical events.

13.   Of the following statements regarding eptifibatide (Integrilin; COR Therapeutics, South San Francisco, CA) treatment, all are TRUE, **EXCEPT:**

    a. It is used concomitantly with heparin and aspirin.
    b. It decreases the rate of death and MI in patients with acute coronary syndromes.
    c. During the infusion the aPTT should be maintained between 50 and 70 seconds.
    d. It is cleared equally by renal and nonrenal mechanisms.
    e. Age is not a contraindication to treatment.

ANSWER: c

The aPTT should be maintained between 50 and 70 seconds unless percutaneous coronary intervention (PCI) is performed. During PCI the ACT should be maintained between 300 and 350 seconds.

In the IMPACT II and PURSUIT studies, eptifibatide was used concomitantly with heparin and aspirin.

The PURSUIT trial included patients presenting with acute coronary syndromes (unstable angina or non Q wave MI).

The IMPACT II trial included patients undergoing percutaneous coronary revascularization. In both trials the use of eptifibatide reduced the incidence of endpoint events early during the treatment and at 30 days.

The drug is equally cleared by renal and nonrenal mechanisms; if creatinine is less than 2.0 mg/dL, the 180 μg/kg bolus and the 2.0 μg/kg/min infusion can be used; if creatinine is 2.0 to 4.0 mg/dL, use a 135 μg/kg bolus and 0.5 μg/kg/min infusion.

Age is not a contraindication to treatment.

14.   Heparin is used routinely during angioplasty to prevent abrupt vessel closure. All of the following are true properties of heparin, **EXCEPT:**

   a. Heparin is able to bind to AT III.
   b. Nonanticoagulant fractions are as effective as the anticoagulant fractions in prevention of neointimal proliferation.
   c. The antiproliferative effect is dose-dependent and greater for low molecular weight heparin (LMWH).
   d. The antiproliferative action is related to incorporation into the cell membrane.

ANSWER: d

Incorporation into the cell nucleus appears to be important in the antiproliferative actions of heparin (*Circulation* 1994;90:908–914).

The anticoagulant and antithrombotic action of heparin is dependent on its binding to AT III, resulting in conformational change that allows AT III to bind avidly with factors IIa and Xa.

Cell culture studies have shown that the nonanticoagulant fractions are as effective as the coagulant fractions in prevention of neointimal proliferation.

The antiproliferative activity is greater for LMWH. The effect is dose-dependent.

15.   The revised labeling for the use of Glucophage in patients with type II diabetes requiring studies using iodinated contrast materials contains all of the following, **EXCEPT:**

   a. Special recommendations pertain only to those cases that require intravascular administration.

b. Current Glucophage treatment is a contraindication to using contrast dye.
c. Glucophage should be withheld for 48 hours after the procedure.
d. Glucophage should be stopped at the time of the procedure.

ANSWER: b

With Glucophage, serious adverse effects are rare and primarily limited to lactic acidosis, a potentially life-threatening condition (half of cases may be fatal). Nearly all cases have been reported in patients with renal insufficiency.

The half-life of Glucophage is 6 hours and it is eliminated through the kidneys.

Glucophage should be stopped at the time of or prior to the angiography, and restarted 48 hours after the procedure if the renal function is normal.

16.   Of the following statements regarding the use of ticlopidine, all are TRUE, **EXCEPT:**

a. It has been associated with thrombotic thrombocytopenic purpura (TTP), a rare complication, with a high mortality rate, that is difficult to predict.
b. The incidence of neutropenia is 2.4%; it is usually reversible when the drug is stopped.
c. It increases serum cholesterol by approximately 8% to 10%.
d. It has a delayed onset of action, making it inappropriate for acute management.

ANSWER: d

Despite its delayed onset of action (usually requires 3 days for full effect), ticlopidine has been used in patients who receive stents; in several studies it was started the day of the procedure without a demonstrable deleterious effect (*N Engl J Med* 1996;334:1084–1089). Often loading doses of 500 mg for the first few days are used.

TTP is a serious complication that has been reported in 60 patients. Since there is a potential benefit to early and aggressive treatment of TTP with plasmapheresis, routine counts are recommended for all patients treated with ticlopidine, and they should be informed of the potential serious hematologic toxicity and the need for monitoring (*Ann Intern Med* 1998;128:541–544).

17.   Of the following statements regarding aspirin, all are TRUE, **EXCEPT:**

    a. It selectively acetylates the hydroxyl group of a serine residue of the platelet prostaglandin G/H synthase 1 (cyclooxygenase), resulting in decrease conversion of arachidonate to ultimately thromboxane A2.

    b. The dose required to almost completely suppress the biosynthesis of thromboxane A2 is 100 mg; this is a cumulative effect, thus lower daily dosages are needed thereafter (usually 30 to 50 mg).

    c. Gastrointestinal bleeding and probably intracranial bleeding are side effects that are dose-dependent.

    d. It decreases the incidence of acute coronary occlusion after angioplasty by 50% when given before the procedure.

    e. Aspirin may enhance some of the beneficial effects of angiotensin-converting inhibitors in patients with ischemic cardiomyopathy and severe congestive heart failure.

ANSWER: e

Aspirin reduces the effect of angiotensin-converting inhibitor on systemic vascular resistance, left ventricular filling pressure, and pulmonary resistance in this subset of patients, probably due inhibition of vasodilator prostaglandins (*N Engl J Med* 1994;330: 1287–1294).

18.   Which one of the following patients should not receive protamine?

    a. A 50-year-old woman with myasthenia gravis.

    b. A 62-year-old woman with end-stage renal disease, on hemodialysis.

    c. A 65-year-old patient whose diabetes is well controlled with neutral protamine Hagedorn (NPH) insulin.

    d. 40-year-old man who has a documented intracranial atrioventricular (AV) malformation.

ANSWER: c

Protamine can reverse the anticoagulant effect of heparin in a dose of approximately 1 mg for every 100 units of heparin.

Protamine is associated with a 2% risk of anaphylaxis or serious hypotensive episodes. The risk of protamine reactions is increased in patients with prior exposure to NPH insulin. Therefore, protamine should not be administered to patients with prior exposure to NPH insulin.

19.   A 55-year-old woman is admitted with unstable angina. She is treated with β-blockers, aspirin, I.V. nitroglycerin, and heparin. Despite maximum medical treat-

ment, she continues to have brief episodes of resting angina; therefore she is referred for coronary angiography, which reveals a 90% stenosis of the mid left anterior descending (LAD) coronary artery. She undergoes percutaneous revascularization and a stent is placed at the site of the stenosis. An excellent result is obtained, with 0% residual stenosis. The patient is discharged home in 48 hours, on β-blockers, aspirin 325 mg by mouth (P.O.), every day (QD), and ticlopidine 250 mg P.O., QD for 2 weeks only. You see her in your office at 2 weeks after her angioplasty; she is symptom-free and plans to return to work next week. Eight days after her last visit, you receive a telephone call from her family and learn that she was admitted emergently to the hospital 2 hours ago with confusion, fever, and a skin rash. You order blood work stat. Which one of the following tests is more likely to be normal?

   a. Hemoglobin
   b. Creatinine
   c. Lactic dehydrogenase (LDH)
   d. PT/PTT

ANSWER: d

The suspected diagnosis is TTP. This patient was taking ticlopidine for 2 weeks and her presentation with skin rash (especially palpable purpura), neurological symptoms, and fever should immediately raise the suspicion of TTP. Ticlopidine is prescribed for less than 1 month in 80% of patients. Most patients with TTP will have low hemoglobin and high LDH due to hemolysis, elevated creatinine levels, and severe thrombocytopenia. However, the coagulation studies are normal. A peripheral blood smear will show polychromasia, stippling, nucleated red cells, and schistocytes (*Cleve Clin J Med* 1998;65:209–214).

20.   Regarding the syndrome that the patient discussed above developed, which one of the following statements is TRUE?

   a. Hemolytic anemia, thrombocytopenia, neurological symptoms, fever, and renal dysfunction represent the pentad of symptoms characterizing the syndrome.
   b. This is an immune process causing platelet destruction.
   c. Closer monitoring of count cell/chemistry would have ensued earlier diagnosis.
   d. Early biopsy of the skin, muscle, and gingiva would have helped in the diagnosis.

ANSWER: a

TTP is a syndrome of disseminated thrombotic occlusions of the microcirculation, with 5 characteristics: hemolytic anemia, thrombocytopenia, neurological symptoms, fever, and renal dysfunction. Only 40% of patients develop the full pentad (*Cleve Clin J Med* 1998;65:209–214).

In TTP, thrombocytopenia develops secondary to a nonimmune mechanism. The mechanism by which ticlopidine induces the clinical manifestations of TTP seems to be related to an altered platelet function. Microthrombi and fibrin networks are laid down in the small vessels. Red blood cells are damaged by these networks and are destroyed in the spleen or the microcirculation. Platelets are either consumed in the microthrombi or damaged and removed by the reticuloendothelial system.

Fever is uncommon initially but invariably develops.

Neurological manifestations including headache, confusion, cranial nerves palsies, seizures, and coma progress rapidly.

Serum creatinine is elevated, but rarely above 1.5 mg/dL.

The onset of ticlopidine-associated TTP is difficult to predict, despite close monitoring of platelet counts (*Ann Intern Med* 1998; 128:541–544).

Biopsy of the skin, muscle, and gingiva has a low diagnostic yield.

Match the following:

21.   Heparin

22.   Hirudin

23.   Argatroban

24.   Integrilin

25.   Tirofiban

    a. Direct inhibitor of thrombin
    b. Indirect inhibitor of thrombin
    c. Fibrinogen receptor antagonist

ANSWERS: 21-b, 22-a, 23-a, 24-c, 25-c

Heparin is a sulfated glycosaminoglycan. Heparin and other indirect thrombin inhibitors (dermatan sulfates, heparin sulfates) inactivate thrombin by avidly binding to AT III. AT III is a protein found along the endothelial cells. In a physiological state, endogenous levels of AT III are able to inhibit the low levels of thrombin and prevent coagulation. A more potent stimulus (ruptured atherosclerotic plaque, for example) will overcome the inactivation effect of AT III and coagulation will proceed. The anticoagulant effect of heparin is severely limited by this dependence on AT III. Furthermore, an endovascular site of injury containing activated platelets is resistant to the effect of heparin due to secretion of platelet factor IV, which blocks the interaction between heparin and AT III. Furthermore, heparin-AT III complex is active only against circulating thrombin and not against thrombin within the clot (*Thromb Haemost* 1997;78[1]:364–366).

Hirudin, hirulog, and argatroban do not require the presence of AT III—they are direct thrombin inhibitors. Hirudin is a polypeptide extracted from the salivary gland of the leech *Hirudo medicinalis,* and is available now in the recombinant form. It does not require the presence of AT III and is not inactivated by platelet factor IV. Hirudin was compared to heparin as adjunctive therapy to tPA for the treatment of acute MI. Although the TIMI 5 pilot trial (*J Am Coll Cardiol* 1994;23:993–1003) showed a reduced rate of in-hospital deaths and reinfarctions with hirudin, the larger TIMI 9 trial (*J Am Coll Cardiol* 1995;25:305–375) failed to show a significant difference between adjunctive heparin and hirudin in acute MI patients treated with thrombolytics. The GUSTO IIA trial (*Circulation* 1994;90:1631–1637) showed that the incidence of hemorrhagic stroke was greater in patients receiving hirudin than in patients receiving heparin. Hirudin was evaluated in patients with unstable angina undergoing PTCA (HELVETICA study; *N Engl J Med* 1995;333:757–763); despite fewer cardiac events in the hirudin group in the first 4 days, there was no difference in the event-free survival at 7 months between heparin- and hirudin-treated patients. The Hirulog Angioplasty Study (*N Engl J Med* 1995;333:764–769) also failed to show any significant difference in cardiac events (death, MI, target vessel revascularization) between the two drugs at 6 months follow-up.

Fibrinogen receptor antagonists can be divided into two large groups: monoclonal antibodies to Gp IIb/IIIa, and competitive antagonists for binding to platelet Gp IIb/IIIa. The monoclonal antibody chimeric 7E3 Fab, largely known as abciximab, will be the main topic of other questions in this manual.

Integrilin competes with fibrinogen for binding to activated Gp IIb/IIIa receptors on the platelet surface. It was evaluated in the PURSUIT study of unstable ischemic syndromes: there was a significant reduction in death, MI, and target vessel revascularization at 24 hours and the effect was maintained at 30 days. Data are positive for its use during PCI, and studies are still ongoing to determine the best dose.

Tirofiban is a peptidomimetic molecule, a competitive antagonist as well, that has shown reductions in death and MI when used in patients with unstable ischemic syndromes. It was also studied in the RESTORE trial (*Circulation* 1996;94:1–5) of high-risk patients undergoing PTCA. At 48 hours, tirofiban therapy was associated with significantly fewer events, but the advantage was not maintained at 30 days.

26.   The term *passivation* refers to:

  a. Switching from a regular balloon to a perfusion balloon in patients with low tolerance for pain, allowing longer balloon inflations.
  b. Performing a percutaneous revascularization procedure on a patient under general anesthesia, mostly in patients who cannot lie flat because of CHF.
  c. The change in an arterial surface from one that supports platelet deposition to one that does not.
  d. A property of a material to be deformed continuously and permanently without rupture (eg, stents).

ANSWER: c

It was shown that a 12-hour infusion after bolus injection of Gp IIb/IIIa inhibitor (abciximab) may promote *passivation* of the vascular intimal surface, thereby exerting long-term antithrombotic effect and reducing the need for repeat angioplasty (*Am J Cardiol* 1995;75:27B-33B).

27.   Of the following statements regarding nitrate therapy, all are TRUE, **EXCEPT:**

  a. They all go extensive first-pass hepatic metabolism when given orally, except the mononitrates.
  b. They ultimately act through liberation of NO by the endothelium.
  c. I.C. nitroglycerin is the drug of choice for "no reflow" phenomena.
  d. Tolerance develops if no daily nitrate-free period is given.

ANSWER: c

A "no reflow" phenomenon can complicate any method of reperfusion, from lytic therapy to angioplasty and rotablation atherectomy. Nitroglycerin does not improve no reflow unless there is superimposed spasm. Although no randomized data are available, the drugs that have been reported to improve impaired flow by I.C. administration are calcium channel blockers (verapamil, diltiazem) or adenosine.

Despite good gastrointestinal absorption, nitrates undergo extensive first-pass hepatic metabolism that have even called into question their therapeutic efficacy. The mononitrates (isosorbide-5-mononitrate) are completely bioavailable and do not have this problem.

The organic nitrates are prodrugs; they biotransform by denitration with the subsequent liberation of NO (previously known as endothelium-derived relaxing factor), which in turn stimulates guanyl cyclase, leading to the conversion of guanosine triphosphate (GTP) to cyclic guanosine monophosphate, which causes vasodilation. The mechanism of denitration remains controversial.

Tolerance is not due to altered pharmacokinetics. Although some loss of hemodynamic effects occurs, some vascular effects persist, plasma volume remains expanded, and withdrawal is associated with a decrease of exercise performance. The mechanism of tolerance remains poorly understood. The only proven method to prevent it is a nitrate-free interval during each 24-hour period (*N Engl J Med* 1998;338:520–531).

28.   All of the following statements regarding the synthetic nonpeptide inhibitors of GpIIb/IIIa receptor are TRUE, **EXCEPT:**

   a. They are reversible antagonists, with a shorter effect than monoclonal antibodies.
   b. They are not immunogenic.
   c. They can be given orally.
   d. They have not yet been tested in humans.

ANSWER: d

The synthetic nonpeptide IIb/IIIa inhibitors are reversible antagonists with a shorter effect than monoclonal antibodies. The effect of Tirofiban is 3 hours, whereas the effect of abciximab is 3 days. They are not immunogenic.

In order for the IIb/IIIa receptor antagonists to be active, they have to inhibit more than 90% of the receptors. Fradafibran, an oral IIb/IIIa receptor antagonist, can block more than 80% of receptors, in a reversible fashion (Braunwald E. *Heart Disease. A Textbook of Cardiovascular Medicine*. Philadelphia: W.B. Saunders Co.; 1997: 1820).

These agents can be administered orally; randomized trials have recently been completed or are under way.

29.   Of the following statements regarding thrombocytopenia in a patient who underwent a coronary artery intervention, all are TRUE, **EXCEPT:**

    a. The rate of thrombocytopenia induced by abciximab (chimeric 7E3 Fab) second administration is 6% to 7%.
    b. The time frame of HIT is different from that of thrombocytopenia induced by readministration of abciximab.
    c. The medical treatment is the same for HIT and abciximab-induced thrombocytopenia.
    d. The platelet count of patients treated with abciximab should be drawn in 3 separate tubes (on citrate, edetic acid [EDTA], and heparin).

ANSWER: b

In the EPIC trial (*N Engl J Med* 1994;330:956–961), the human antichimeric antibody (HACA) formation rate was 6.5%; chimeric 7E3 Fab was specifically engineered to reduce antigenicity. The preliminary data show that readministration of abciximab in HACA-negative patients is safe and effective. There are no data regarding the patients who developed HACA upon initial abciximab administration and who require additional treatment with abciximab. The most likely complication, if any, may be an immune-related thrombocytopenia.

HIT may appear in two forms: type I HIT is a mild, self-limited thrombocytopenia, and type II HIT is a severe syndrome characterized by thrombocytopenia and frequent thromboembolic complications from platelet thrombi. The treatment for type II HIT is to stop the heparin and give oral anticoagulants and thrombolytic agents. HIT usually develops after 5 or more days of therapy (or much sooner in patients previously exposed to heparin). Most cases of thrombocytopenia associated with abciximab usually occur in the first 24 hours of therapy and are not related to HACA development. Attention should be paid to cases of abciximab readministration, when thrombocytopenia can develop in the first 24 hours but also in the following 4 to 5 days; hence, the platelet level should be checked in this group of patients 4 to 5 days following readministration. Thrombocytopenia associated with abciximab therapy can be corrected as clinically indicated, with platelet transfusion.

In patients treated with abciximab, the platelet count should be drawn in 3 separate tubes with one tube containing EDTA, one citrate, and one heparin to exclude pseudothrombocytopenia due to in vitro anticoagulant reaction. A peripheral blood smear should also be obtained.

30. The use of thrombolytic therapy in the setting of angioplasty performed for unstable angina is:

    a. Strongly indicated because of the presence of thrombus, frequently present in unstable coronary syndromes.
    b. Indicated only in cases in which dissection and thrombus are evident on angiography.
    c. Not indicated because, in association with heparin, the risk of bleeding increases prohibitively.
    d. Not generally indicated because of poorer outcome.

ANSWER: d

It is largely accepted today that the thrombolytic therapy (tPA, urokinase) used as an adjunctive to angioplasty for unstable angina negatively influences the outcome. The TAUSA trial (Thrombolysis and Angioplasty in Unstable Angina; *Circulation* 1994;90:69–77) showed that prophylactic administration of urokinase I.C. is associated with increased occurrence of clinical endpoints of recurrent ischemia, MI, and emergent bypass surgery (12.9% versus 6.3%; $P<0.02$). The outcome was worse in patients with unstable angina than in patients with post-MI angina.

In the TIMI IIIB trial (*Circulation* 1994;89:1545–1556) patients with unstable angina and non Q wave MI who received tPA plus heparin had a higher occurrence of fatal and nonfatal MI at 42 days after presentation (7.4%) as opposed to patients treated only with heparin and angioplasty (4.9%; $P=0.06$).The explanation for these results resides in the dual action of thrombolytic agents: clot-dissolving and procoagulant effect.

Thrombolytics expose the fibrin-associated thrombin, which stimulates thrombosis. They also activate platelets directly. In unstable angina, the coronary thrombus is platelet rich. The presence of intimal dissection may further compromise the situation by producing mural thrombus with subsequent luminal occlusion.

Match the following:

31.   tPA

32.   Streptokinase

33.   Urokinase

34.   Reteplase

    a. Binds to plasminogen and then activates it
    b. Cleaves a peptide bond of plasminogen, activating it

ANSWERS: 31-b, 32-a, 33-b, 34-b

tPA is a naturally occurring enzyme; it is a serine protease that cleaves plasminogen. It also has a binding site for fibrin that allows it to attach to a formed thrombus preferentially and lyse it; however, some degree of systemic plasminogen activation occurs. The dose is 100 mg (15 mg I.V. bolus, with the remainder over 90 minutes), and the plasma half-life is 4 to 8 minutes. (*N Engl J Med* 1993;329:703–709).

Reteplase is a deletion mutant of tPA with a longer half-life (15 minutes) and lower fibrin specificity. It is given as two 10-international unit (IU) boluses 30 minutes apart. It is as effective as tPA. (*Circulation* 1998;97:1632–1646).

TNK-tPA is another mutant of tPA with a longer half-life (20 minutes), increased fibrin specificity, and resistance to plasminogen activator inhibitor-1. It produces similar TIMI III flow at 90 minutes to tPA.

Streptokinase binds to plasminogen in a 1:1 ratio, causing a change in molecular conformation so that the complex becomes an active enzyme that in turn cleaves a peptide bond in other plasminogen molecules to activate them. It is antigenic and should not be readministered within a few years of treatment. The dose is 1.5 million units administered over 1 hour. The plasma half-life is 15 to 25 minutes.

Urokinase directly cleaves plasminogen in a fashion similar to tPA. Its half-life is 15 to 20 minutes and the dose is a 1 million unit I.V. bolus followed by 1 million units over 1 hour.

35. Of the following medical therapies, which one is correct for the treatment of contrast-dye–related anaphylactic shock?

    a. Draw 1 mL of 1:1000 epinephrine, and dilute it to a total volume of 10 mL (10 µg/mL). Then administer it I.V., 1 mL every (Q) 1 minute, until BP is restored.
    b. Administer boluses of 10 µg of epinephrine Q 1 minute until the desired BP is obtained, and continue with an I.V. infusion of 1 to 4 µg/min to maintain the BP at the desired level.
    c. Administer 0.3 cc of 1:1000 solution subcutaneously (S.Q.) Q 15 minutes up to 1 mL.
    d. Rapid administration of 1 mg I.V. of epinephrine will restore the BP in 90% of cases.

ANSWER: b

The guidelines for management of anaphylactoid reactions in the cardiac catheterization laboratory (*Cathet Cardiovasc Diagn* 1995; 34:99–104) are the following:

- In case of moderate to severe facial and laryngeal edema as well as in cases of anaphylactic shock, epinephrine should be administered intravenously.
- The preparation of epinephrine for I.V. administration is as follows: 1 cc of 1:10,000 solution (which contains 0.1 mg/cc or 100 µg/cc) will be diluted in 10 cc resulting in a solution of 10 µg/cc.

- The correct and the only accepted mode of administration of epinephrine for the above mentioned conditions is the one described in answer b.
- Urticaria and skin itching, moderate bronchospasm, and mild facial and mild laryngeal edema can be treated with S.Q. epinephrine as depicted in answer c.

36.   Of the following statements regarding adjunctive therapy for stents, all are FALSE, **EXCEPT:**

a. The treatment with aspirin and ticlopidine has comparable impact on stent thrombosis to that with aspirin and warfarin, but has less bleeding complications.
b. Warfarin therapy should be used as an adjunctive medication only in cases of suboptimal stent deployment.
c. Prophylactic antibiotic therapy should be used according to the same criteria employed for valvular diseases.
d. If a patient is allergic/intolerant to ticlopidine, clopidogrel can be used instead.

ANSWER: d

A randomized trial (STARS) compared aspirin, aspirin plus ticlopidine, and aspirin plus warfarin as adjunctive therapy to successfully implanted Palmaz-Schatz stents; there was a 2- to 5-fold reduction in the rate of acute ischemic complications in patients treated with aspirin plus ticlopidine (*Circulation* 1996; 94:I685).

The use of aspirin plus ticlopidine after high-risk stenting was associated with 7- to 10-fold decrease in stent thrombosis and acute ischemic complications implicitly, as well as bleeding complications (ISAR study; *N Engl J Med* 1996;334:1084–1089).

Although there is not a consensus regarding antibiotic prophylaxis for patients who received a stent, many physicians recommend the use of prophylaxis until the stent is fully endothelialized; each case should be evaluated individually.

Clopidogrel is a new antiplatelet drug that can be used instead of ticlopidine. There are no randomized studies comparing use of the two drugs in poststent management. The CAPRIE study (*Lancet* 1996;348:1329–1339) showed that clopidogrel can be used to reduce atherosclerotic events (MI, stroke, and vascular death).

Match the following:

37.   Ticlopidine

38.   Aspirin

39.   Clopidogrel

40.   Tirofiban

    a. Inhibits thromboxane formation.
    b. Inhibits adenosine diphosphate- (ADP) mediated activation of the GpIIb/IIIa complex.
    c. Nonprotein reversible antagonist of the platelet GpIIb/IIIa receptor.

ANSWERS: 37-b, 38-a, 39-b, 40-c

Aspirin, ticlopidine, clopidogrel and tirofiban are inhibitors of platelet function.

Aspirin selectively inhibits thromboxane formation but only partially inhibits the platelet aggregation induced by ADP, collagen, or thrombin.

Ticlopidine and Clopidogrel are noncompetitive but selective antagonists of ADP-induced platelet aggregation by blocking Gp IIb/IIIa activation.

Tirofiban is a synthetic IIb/IIIa inhibitor. The effect is short (3 hours compared to 3 days for abciximab). It is not immunogenic.

41.   Which of the following is recommended for the use of heparin after PTCA?
    a. Discontinue immediately.
    b. Continue at full strength for an additional 6 to 12 hours.
    c. Continue at full strength for 24 hours, during sheath removal use half-strength.

ANSWER: a

There are few data regarding the use of heparin post procedure, and small randomized data fail to support the use of heparin for 12 to 24 hours as a way to reduce ischemic complications (*J Am Coll Cardiol* 1994;24:1214–1219). However, these studies excluded vessels with suboptimal results, major dissections, thrombus, or patients post MI.

Furthermore, the use of antiplatelet therapy (like abciximab) has reduced the heparin need even more. The fear of acute/subacute stent thrombosis is best avoided by adequate stent deployment and adjuvant antiplatelet therapy.

Sheath removal is best done as soon as the ACT is below 175 seconds, which can sometimes be immediately postprocedure when abciximab is used.

42.   Patients with history of HIT who are to undergo angioplasty may receive instead all of the following, **EXCEPT:**

  a. LMWH
  b. Hirudin
  c. Bivalirudin (Hirulog)
  d. Abciximab

ANSWER: a

LMWH may cross-react and should not be used in these patients.

Bivalirudin, a synthetic derivative of hirudin, inhibits both clot-bound and free thrombin. It has been used in patients undergoing angioplasty for unstable angina (postinfarction) and, compared to heparin (*N Engl J Med* 1995;333:764–769), it did not reduce death, abrupt vessel closure, or infarction but had a better safety profile in terms of major bleeding; hence, it is an acceptable alternative.

It is reasonable to use abciximab as adjunctive therapy as well.

Hirudin was studied in the HELVETICA trial (*N Engl J Med* 1995;333:757–763); again, no reductions in clinical events or

restenosis were seen at 6 months, despite reductions in major cardiac events at 4 days.

43.   Which one of the following measures reduces restenosis after PTCA in
small coronary arteries (diameter <2.5 mm)?

    a. High-dose multivitamins
    b. Probucol
    c. High-dose multivitamins combined with probucol
    d. Stenting

ANSWER: b

Oxidative stress after PTCA appears to be an important contributor to restenosis. Oxidized LDL produces endothelial dysfunction
and activation of macrophages, resulting in the release of growth
factors conductive to rapid tissue production. Probucol has powerful antioxidant properties, limiting neointimal formation and
the vascular remodeling involved in restenosis (Probucol Angioplasty Restenosis Trial. *J Am Coll Cardiol* 1997;30:855). Probucol
inhibits the secretion of interleukin-1 by macrophages, reducing
the production of matrix metalloproteinases by smooth muscle
cells.

High-dose multivitamins have failed to reduce restenosis (*N Engl
J Med* 1997;337:365).

Use of probucol alone resulted in better results than the combination of probucol and high-dose vitamins; it is possible that
high-dose multivitamins paradoxically act as pro-oxidants.

High-dose lovastatin does not reduce restenosis (*N Engl J Med*
1994;331:1331).

No studies have definitively demonstrated that stenting of arteries with a diameter less than 2.7 mm reduces restenosis.

44.   Of the following statements regarding coronary vasodilatation, all are
TRUE, **EXCEPT:**

    a. Nitroglycerin I.C. has a more predictive response than sublingual (S.L.)
       or I.V. nitroglycerin.
    b. Ionic contrast agents may induce vasodilatation up to 20%.

c. Nonionic contrast agents produce more vasodilatation than ionic agents.
d. The effect of I.C. nitroglycerin peaks at 1 minute.

ANSWER: c

Nonionic contrast agents produce only minimal vasodilatation, not exceeding 6%.

45.   Which one of the following statements is TRUE regarding the aspirin/ticlopidine (A/T) combination compared to aspirin/warfarin (A/W) combination?

a. A/T results in less bleeding complications but higher in-stent acute thrombosis.
b. A/T results in less bleeding complications and less in-stent thrombosis.
c. A/T combination results in the same clinical outcome provided the warfarin is given to maintain an international normalized ratio (INR) above 3.0.
d. There are no data to support the benefit of one therapy over the other.

ANSWER: b

There are compelling data to support the use of A/T combination after stent placement in order to decrease the risk of bleeding and in-stent thrombosis.

46.   Of the following statements regarding aspirin allergy, all are TRUE, **EX-CEPT:**

a. Patients with asthma and rhino-sinusitis may develop aspirin sensitivity.
b. Desensitization involves administering progressively higher doses of aspirin at specific time intervals.
c. Patients with aspirin-induced angio-edema, urticaria, or anaphylaxis should not undergo desensitization.
d. A cutaneous reaction to aspirin puts the patient at risk for anaphylaxis upon readministration of the drug.
e. A patient who underwent successful desensitization but interrupted his or her aspirin for 3 days during a hiking trip requires a new desensitization attempt.

ANSWER: d

Patients who had a cutaneous reaction to aspirin are not at increased risk of anaphylaxis when the drug is readministered. H1 and H2 blockers can control the symptoms.

Up to 30% of patients with asthma and rhino-sinusitis may develop aspirin allergy.

Desensitization involves the oral administration of progressively higher doses of aspirin, at specific time intervals; this will result in a refractory period during which aspirin can be safely given. The desensitization period can be maintained as long as aspirin treatment is not interrupted.

Chapter 4

Instrumentation and Techniques

QUESTIONS

Match the following angiographic views with the corresponding coronary artery segments:

1.   60° left anterior oblique (LAO)/25° caudal

2.   30° right anterior oblique (RAO)/20° cranial

3.   30° RAO/25° caudal

4.   60° LAO/25° cranial

    a.   Proximal left main (LM), proximal LAD, proximal LCX.
    b.   LCX and marginal branches.
    c.   Mid and distal LAD and diagonal branches.
    d.   Mid right coronary artery (RCA), the origin and course of patent ductus arteriosus (PDA).

5.   In what view is dominance most easily assessed?

    a.   LAO caudal
    b.   LAO cranial
    c.   RAO caudal
    d.   Shallow RAO

6.   Of the following statements regarding the angiography of left coronary system when the LM coronary artery is absent, all are TRUE, **EXCEPT:**

    a.   Generally, the LAD has a more anterior origin than the LCX.
    b.   When the LAD has an anterior take off, it can be engaged with the left Judkins catheter with counter-clockwise rotation.
    c.   A catheter with a larger curve is useful to selectively engage the LAD in this setting.
    d.   A catheter with a shorter curve tends to engage selectively in LAD.

85

7.   Which is/are the best view(s) to confirm coaxial alignment between the catheter tip and LM?

    a.   50° LAO/30° caudal or 5° RAO/20° caudal
    b.   30° LAO/50° cranial
    c.   30° RAO
    d.   10° RAO/50° cranial or 90° LAO

8.   Of the following statements regarding balloon compliance, all are FALSE, **EXCEPT:**

    a.   There is a direct relationship between compliance and stretchability.
    b.   Compliance is defined as the ability of a balloon to adapt to the shape of a vessel.
    c.   Compliance refers to the tendency of an angioplasty balloon to enlarge after sequential inflations at the same pressure.
    d.   Compliant balloons are associated with higher burst pressures and are useful in rigid lesions that cannot be dilated at inflation pressures <10 atm.

9.   Underestimation of coronary artery disease (CAD) severity can be due to all of the following, **EXCEPT:**

    a.   Diffuse atherosclerotic narrowing
    b.   Inadequate angiographic projections
    c.   Distal obstruction
    d.   Poststenotic dilatation
    e.   Concentric, discrete stenosis

10.   Of the following statements regarding IVUS, all are TRUE, **EXCEPT:**

    a.   Current catheters have distal tips of 0.9 to 1.7 mm in diameter; therefore only vessels with a diameter >0.9 mm can be visualized.
    b.   The higher the frequency used, the more attenuation and backscatter from red blood cells and reduced penetration.

c. The complication rate is about 1.1% (spasm, wire entrapment, and dissection).
d. The internal lamina elastica is a weak reflector of ultrasound waves.
e. The sensitivity for the detection of thrombus is low and for calcium is high.

11.   Which of the following is TRUE regarding CFR when measured with a Doppler flow wire?

a. It may be low in patients with normal coronary arteries by angiogram and IVUS.
b. Non–endothelium-dependent vasodilation function is measured with infusions of acetylcholine and nitroglycerin.
c. Endothelium-dependent vasodilation function of the resistance arteries is measured with adenosine.
d. Left ventricular hypertrophy and hypertension do not reduce CFR.

12.   If X is diameter stenosis, Y is immediate postprocedure diameter, and Z is late follow-up diameter stenosis, which one of the following best expresses the late loss?

a. $Y - X$
b. $Y - Z$
c. $Y - Z/Y - X$
d. $X + Y - Z$

13.   The "acute gain" refers to:

a. The difference between minimal lumen diameter (MLD) before the procedure and maximal luminal diameter of a normal segment in the same artery.
b. The difference between MLD before and after the intervention.
c. First balloon inflation followed by <50% residual stenosis, without dissection or distal embolization.
d. The difference between maximum and MLD immediately after intervention.

14.   Of the following statements regarding aorto-ostial lesions on SVGs, all are TRUE, **EXCEPT:**

    a. They have high restenosis rates.
    b. They are often rigid, with suboptimal balloon results.
    c. Debulking is often necessary, usually with rotational atherectomy (small burrs).
    d. Optimal stent placement requires that 1 mm of stent protrudes into the aorta.
    e. IVUS is contraindicated.

15.   The two physical principles at the basis of rotablation system operation are:

    a. "Differential cutting" and "thermal effect."
    b. "Microcavitation" and "thermal effect."
    c. "Differential cutting" and "orthogonal displacement of friction."
    d. "Orthogonal displacement of friction" and "microcavitation."

16.   With regard to the guide catheter selection when performing a rotational atherectomy, all of the following statements are TRUE, **EXCEPT:**

    a. Significant support or deep intubation is extremely important when performing rotational atherectomy.
    b. The guide catheter inner diameter should be 0.004″ larger than the largest burr used.
    c. Guider catheters with side holes are generally recommended.
    d. Coaxial alignment is of paramount importance.

17.   Of the following statements regarding coronary thrombus, all are FALSE, **EXCEPT:**

    a. Transluminal extraction catheter atherectomy eliminates the "no reflow" phenomenon or distal embolization.
    b. Rotablation atherectomy can be used in certain cases of coronary stenosis associated with angiographically visible thrombus.

c. The insertion of stents in vessels with diameter <2.5 mm has been associated with increased mortality rate secondary to abrupt closure.

d. Once coronary thrombus is present, the risk of distal embolization and no reflow is almost equal in native vessels and in vein grafts.

18.   Which one of the following statements regarding coronary artery perforations is TRUE?

a. In treating class I and II coronary perforations, reversal of heparin anticoagulation is usually sufficient.

b. Aspirin and heparin should be stopped in all cases of coronary perforation.

c. Regardless of the device used for coronary revascularization, the risk of perforation is increased when complex lesion morphology is present (angulated segment, total occlusion, bifurcation).

d. Balloon rupture is not associated with coronary artery perforation.

19.   Which one of the following patients is less likely to develop contrast-induced nephropathy?

a. A 75-year-old man admitted with 4 days history of diarrhea.

b. A 55-year-old with recent diagnosed multiple myeloma.

c. A 39-year-old with history of cirrhosis.

d. A 55-year-old woman with history of minimal change glomerulonephritis 20 years ago and a creatinine of 1.1 mg/dL.

Match the following contrast agents used in coronary angiograpy:

20.   These substances dissociate into cations and iodine-containing anions.

21.   These substances go into solutions as single neutral molecules.

22.   These substances contain calcium-chelating properties.

23.   The osmolality of these agents is 600 to 900 mOsm/kg as compared to the osmolality of human plasma of 300 mOsm/kg.

    a. Monomeric ionic contrast agents
    b. Nonionic, low-osmolality contrast agents

Regarding TIMI frame count, match the following:

24.   Initial frame

25.   The flow in this vessel is usually slower (on average 1.7 times)

26.   Distal landmark for the RCA

27.   Distal landmark for the LCX

28.   Distal landmark for the LAD

    a. First branch arising from the RCA after the origin of the PDA, regardless of its size
    b. Distal PDA
    c. Most distal branch of the LAD ("whale's tail")
    d. First frame in which the contrast fully enters the artery
    e. Distal AV groove circumflex
    f. Longest marginal branch beyond the lesion
    g. LAD
    h. RCA

29.   Regarding stenting of venous graft lesions, which statement is TRUE?

    a. Balloon angioplasty of venous graft lesions has similar clinical outcome as stenting.
    b. The radial force is not important in stenting venous graft lesions, as the elastic recoil is minimal.

   c. Directional atherectomy provides similar or better effi-
      cacy than stents for vein graft disease.
   d. The outcome of the stent implantation is not dependent
      upon the age of the conduit.

30.   When approaching a left IMA graft for revascularization, all of the following considerations are TRUE, **EXCEPT:**

   a. Use of 60° LAO projection is useful when the subclavian artery is tortuous.
   b. There is a high rate of distal embolization, associated with "no reflow."
   c. A right Judkins catheter can be used.
   d. Pretreatment with nitroglycerin and calcium channel blockers is indicated.

31.   Stenting is indicated in all of the following situations, **EXCEPT:**

   a. Ulcerated lesions
   b. High eccentricity
   c. Intraluminal thrombus
   d. Total occlusion
   e. Highly calcified lesions

32.   True bifurcational lesions (stenosis >50% involving the main vessel and the ostium of its side branch), can be treated with:

   a. Rotational atherectomy followed by balloon inflation
   b. Directional atherectomy followed by balloon inflation
   c. Balloon angioplasty alone
   d. Rotational atherectomy followed by stenting
   e. All of the above

33.   The usual dose of heparin required for coronary angioplasty is:

   a. 10,000 units initially, and 1000 units every hour thereafter
   b. 70 U/kg of weight
   c. 100 U/kg of weight
   d. 15,000 units

Match the following:

34.   Seventy-five percent lesion in mid LAD with 60% lesion at the ostium of second diagonal branch, which is a 2.2 mm diameter vessel originating from the LAD lesion.

35.   Eighty percent proximal LAD with a 1.5 mm diameter first diagonal branch whose ostium has a 70% stenosis.

36.   Eighty percent proximal LCX at the take off of an obtuse marginal branch which has a diameter of 2.2 mm.

37.   Ninety percent mid LAD with a 2.7 mm diameter diagonal that arises immediately beyond the lesion and is free of disease.

    a. Side-branch protection recommended
    b. Side-branch protection not recommended

38.   Of the following statements regarding the left lateral projection, all are TRUE, **EXCEPT:**

    a. The mid portion of the RCA can be seen well without the excessive motion of a straight RAO view.
    b. The anastomosis of left IMA (LIMA) to mid or distal LAD is seen very well in this view.
    c. Proximal and distal LAD and proximal LCX can be well visualized.
    d. The LM ostium can be frequently seen in this projection.

Match each of the following anatomic variants with the appropriate guider catheter:

39.   RCA superior orientation ("shepherd's crook")

40.   RCA inferior orientation

41.   Tortuous LCX

    a.   Hockey stick
    b.   Extra back-up (EBU)
    c.   Multipurpose
    d.   Castillo

Match each of the following clinical situations with its appropriate measure:

42.   Good torque control

43.   Increased flexibility

44.   Kink-resistant

45.   Good support and trackability

    a.   Unicore guidewires
    b.   Floppy guidewires/stainless steel wires
    c.   Glidewires/nitinol wires

46.   Of the following statements regarding stent deployment failure, all are TRUE, **EXCEPT:**

    a.   Proximal vessel tortuosity and/or calcification are associated with increased risk of stent dislodgement.
    b.   In certain circumstances, automatic power injection can be used to deploy a stent.
    c.   Stent embolization, although annoying, is harmless.
    d.   Occasionally, emergency CABG is necessary.

47.   Stenting can safely be used in the following situations:

    a.   SVGs
    b.   Long lesions (>15 mm)
    c.   Acute closure
    d.   Prior restenosis

    e. Chronic total occlusions
    f. a, c, d
    g. a, b, c, d, e

48.   Stenting of small vessels (<3.0 mm in diameter) reduces restenosis.

    a. True
    b. False

Match the following stents:

49.   Multi-Link

50.   Wiktor

51.   Radius

52.   GFX

    a. Slotted-tube
    b. Mesh (self-expanding)
    c. Coil
    d. "Hybrid"

53.   Which of the following is not associated with complications during rotational atherectomy?

    a. Decelerations >5000 rpm
    b. Higher platform rpm
    c. Short runs
    d. Duration of decelerations >10 seconds

54.   Intracoronary administration of thrombolytics is an effective therapy for acute coronary syndromes and the presence of thrombus by angiography.

    a. True
    b. False

55. Of the following statements regarding pacemaker use during rotablation atherectomy procedure, all are TRUE, **EXCEPT:**

    a. Pacemaker should be used when treating ostial LAD, ostial RCA, or ostial LCX.
    b. Temporary pacemaker is recommended when rotablation of RCA or dominant LCX is performed.
    c. Use of large burrs may be associated with AV block and therefore need for temporary pacemaker.
    d. Use of abciximab has significantly decreased the need for temporary pacemaker insertion during rotablation atherectomy.

56. Of the following statements regarding excimer laser coronary atherectomy (ELCA), all are TRUE, **EXCEPT:**

    a. The excimer laser emits pulsed infrared laser light at 308 nm.
    b. Saline infusion technique has allowed a decrease in rate of acute complications related to ELCA.
    c. Once dissection is present, the increase in laser energy can be dangerous.
    d. Bifurcation lesions, highly eccentric lesions, and uncrossable total occlusions are contraindications to ELCA use.

57. Of the following statements regarding IVUS, all are TRUE, **EXCEPT:**

    a. It uses frequencies of 20 to 40 MHz.
    b. Synthetic phased array devices are more flexible and have better guidewire tracking than mechanical devices.
    c. Optimal stent deployment criteria by IVUS includes stent symmetry (symmetry index >0.7), absence of echo-free space between the stent and the wall, adequate cross-sectional area (CSA) ratio of stent to reference vessel greater than 0.8, and no edge tear.
    d. Septals and diagonal branches are indistinguishable when IVUS of the LAD is performed.

Match the following:

58.   Luminal vessel detail

59.   Clot versus dissection

60.   Functional evaluation of a stenosis

61.   Diffuse disease

62.   Arterial wall and vessel dimension

    a.   Doppler wire
    b.   IVUS
    c.   Angioscopy

63.   Of the following statements regarding rotablation atherectomy, all are TRUE, **EXCEPT:**

    a.   Rotational speed fall >5000 rpm below the platform speed allows generation of heat, large particles, and endoluminal trauma.
    b.   Any 0.014″ guiding wire can be used for rotablation, as long as it has a length of >300 cm.
    c.   The internal diameter of the guiding catheter should be 0.004″ larger than the burr diameter.
    d.   The rotablation burr is diamond-coated only on the leading half.

64.   Of the following statements regarding "dynaglide" during rotational atherectomy, all are TRUE, **EXCEPT:**

    a.   It provides 50,000 to 90,000 rpm rotation when the burr is removed from the patient.
    b.   If the "dynaglide" light does not switch off upon deactivation of the dynaglide mode, there may be low gas pressure in the gas tank.
    c.   Wireclip (torque device) should be kept on the wire during "dynaglide."
    d.   If the vessel is small (<2.0 mm), the lesion can be crossed with "dynaglide."

65.   Of the following statements regarding DCA, all are TRUE, **EXCEPT:**

     a.   Distal cutters are available in 5F, 6F, and 7F sizes.
     b.   Guiding catheters for the LCA are available in 10F and 11F, and for the RCA, 9.5F and 10F only.
     c.   Small arteries (2.5 mm), moderate to heavy calcification, proximal angulation >45°, length >20 mm, extensive dissection, and degenerative SVG are all considered unfavorable for DCA.
     d.   The cutter window is 10 mm and opens over a 120° arch.
     e.   The balloon is attached to the opposite of the window and is designed for high-pressure inflations that will securely anchor it in position during cutting.

66.   Of the following statements regarding TEC atherectomy, all are TRUE, **EXCEPT:**

     a.   Any 9F guider catheter can be used as long as good alignment is obtained.
     b.   The TEC guidewire can be used to cross the lesion.
     c.   The cutter must be activated proximal to the lesion and advanced slowly to achieve continuous blood flow in the vacuum bottle.
     d.   Dissection is frequently seen after TEC atherectomy.

67.   The origin of the term LASER is:

     a.   The name of the French physicist who discovered it.
     b.   Light amplification by stimulated emission of radiation.
     c.   Light activity on atherosclerotic plaque, excision, and removal.
     d.   Light activity system/excimer radiation.

68.   Of the following statements regarding the excimer laser ablation, all are TRUE, **EXCEPT:**

     a.   For lesions that are noncalcified and resistant to ablation, increase *fluence* first.

    b. For lesions that are calcified and resistant, increase *repetition rate.*

    c. For lesions that are noncalcified and resistant to ablation, increase *repetition rate* first.

    d. In treating resistant bypass graft lesions, increase in both *fluence* and *repetition rate* can be used.

ANSWERS

1. 60° left anterior oblique (LAO)/25° caudal

2. 30° right anterior oblique (RAO)/20° cranial

3. 30° RAO/25° caudal

4. 60° LAO/25° cranial

    a. Proximal left main (LM), proximal LAD, proximal LCX.
    b. LCX and marginal branches.
    c. Mid and distal LAD and diagonal branches.
    d. Mid right coronary artery (RCA), the origin and course of patent ductus arteriosus (PDA).

ANSWERS: 1-a, 2-c, 3-b, 4-d

5. In what view is dominance most easily assessed?

    a. LAO caudal
    b. LAO cranial
    c. RAO caudal
    d. Shallow RAO

ANSWER: b

The dominant vessel is the one that supplies the posterior diaphragmatic portion of the interventricular septum and the diaphragmatic surface of the left ventricle. The RCA is dominant in 85% of cases. Dominance is most easily assessed in the LAO cranial view.

6. Of the following statements regarding the angiography of left coronary system when the LM coronary artery is absent, all are TRUE, **EXCEPT:**

    a. Generally, the LAD has a more anterior origin than the LCX.
    b. When the LAD has an anterior take off, it can be engaged with the left Judkins catheter with counter-clockwise rotation.
    c. A catheter with a larger curve is useful to selectively engage the LAD in this setting.
    d. A catheter with a shorter curve tends to engage selectively in LAD.

ANSWER: c

In this situation, the origin of LAD is more anterior and superior (and it will be selectively engaged with a left Judkins 3.5) as opposed to the LCX course, which is downward and it will be selectively engaged with a left Judkins 5.0.

7.   Which is/are the best view(s) to confirm coaxial alignment between the catheter tip and LM?

    a. 50° LAO/30° caudal or 5° RAO/20° caudal
    b. 30° LAO/50° cranial
    c. 30° RAO
    d. 10° RAO/50° cranial or 90° LAO

ANSWER: a

The best views to evaluate the alignment of catheter tip/LM are 50° LAO/30° caudal (spider view) and shallow RAO/20° caudal.

8.   Of the following statements regarding balloon compliance, all are FALSE, **EXCEPT:**

    a. There is a direct relationship between compliance and stretchability.
    b. Compliance is defined as the ability of a balloon to adapt to the shape of a vessel.
    c. Compliance refers to the tendency of an angioplasty balloon to enlarge after sequential inflations at the same pressure.
    d. Compliant balloons are associated with higher burst pressures and are useful in rigid lesions that cannot be dilated at inflation pressures <10 atm.

ANSWER: a

Balloon *compliance* is the change in balloon diameter per atmosphere of inflation pressure. Compliance is an index of balloon stretchability. Polyolefin copolymer (POC) balloons have a compliance of 0.095 mm/atm and are generally considered more compliant. Polyethylene terephthalate (PET) balloons have a compliance of 0.010 mm/atm and are less compliant. Cumulative data have shown that there is no difference in angiographic results or ischemic complications between the two types of balloons. Regardless of the compliance, the most important factor in minimizing the risk of dissection, abrupt closure, and major ischemic complications is the accurate balloon sizing (ideal balloon/artery ratio = 0.9 to 1.1).

The ability of a balloon to adapt to the shape of a vessel is called *conformability;* in angulated lesions, more conformable and non-compliant balloons have better angiographic results.

"Creep" refers to the tendency of a balloon to enlarge after sequential inflations at the same pressure. More compliant balloons are associated with more creep.

Noncompliant balloons are associated with higher burst pressures.

9.   Underestimation of coronary artery disease (CAD) severity can be due to all of the following, **EXCEPT:**

    a. Diffuse atherosclerotic narrowing
    b. Inadequate angiographic projections
    c. Distal obstruction
    d. Poststenotic dilatation
    e. Concentric, discrete stenosis

ANSWER: d

Poststenotic dilatation and vasospasm may result in overestimation of CAD (*Circulation* 1996;94:2662–2666).

10.   Of the following statements regarding IVUS, all are TRUE, **EXCEPT:**

    a. Current catheters have distal tips of 0.9 to 1.7 mm in diameter; therefore only vessels with a diameter >0.9 mm can be visualized.
    b. The higher the frequency used, the more attenuation and backscatter from red blood cells and reduced penetration.
    c. The complication rate is about 1.1% (spasm, wire entrapment, and dissection).
    d. The internal lamina elastica is a weak reflector of ultrasound waves.
    e. The sensitivity for the detection of thrombus is low and for calcium is high.

ANSWER: d

The typical IVUS cross-sectional image has a 3-layered appearance: a bright inner layer (*internal elastica lamina*) due to the strong reflection of collagen and elastin, an echolucent second layer (*media*), and a bright outer third layer (*external elastica lamina* and *adventitia*).

11.   Which of the following is TRUE regarding CFR when measured with a Doppler flow wire?

    a. It may be low in patients with normal coronary arteries by angiogram and IVUS.
    b. Non–endothelium-dependent vasodilation function is measured with infusions of acetylcholine and nitroglycerin.
    c. Endothelium-dependent vasodilation function of the resistance arteries is measured with adenosine.
    d. Left ventricular hypertrophy and hypertension do not reduce CFR.

ANSWER: a

Altered coronary vasomotor tone can be found in normal coronary arteries.

Acetylcholine and nitroglycerin are *endothelium-dependent* vasodilators.

Adenosine is an *endothelium-independent* vasodilator.

Left ventricular hypertrophy and hypertension will typically reduce CFR due to the disparity of microcirculation/ventricular mass.

12.   If X is diameter stenosis, Y is immediate postprocedure diameter, and Z is late follow-up diameter stenosis, which one of the following best expresses the late loss?

    a. Y − X
    b. Y − Z
    c. Y − Z/Y − X
    d. X + Y − Z

ANSWER: b

Y − Z = late loss.

Y − X = acute gain.

Y − Z/Y − X = the loss index.

13.   The "acute gain" refers to:

    a.   The difference between minimal lumen diameter (MLD) before the procedure and maximal luminal diameter of a normal segment in the same artery.
    b.   The difference between MLD before and after the intervention.
    c.   First balloon inflation followed by <50% residual stenosis, without dissection or distal embolization.
    d.   The difference between maximum and MLD immediately after intervention.

ANSWER: b

Acute gain is defined as the difference in lumen diameter before and immediately after intervention, and is due to plaque removal and/or arterial expansion.

14.   Of the following statements regarding aorto-ostial lesions on SVGs, all are TRUE, **EXCEPT:**

    a.   They have high restenosis rates.
    b.   They are often rigid, with suboptimal balloon results.
    c.   Debulking is often necessary, usually with rotational atherectomy (small burrs).
    d.   Optimal stent placement requires that 1 mm of stent protrudes into the aorta.
    e.   IVUS is contraindicated.

ANSWER: e

Most interventionalists agree that this particular lesion must be stented.

IVUS is not contraindicated in aorto-ostial lesions. IVUS pre procedure may indicate the need for debulking if calcium is present, in order to allow full stent expansion; IVUS will also assess optimal stent deployment. Use of IVUS may reduce the high restenosis rates seen in most observational studies.

15.   The two physical principles at the basis of rotablation system operation are:

    a.   "Differential cutting" and "thermal effect."
    b.   "Microcavitation" and "thermal effect."
    c.   "Differential cutting" and "orthogonal displacement of friction."
    d.   "Orthogonal displacement of friction" and "microcavitation."

ANSWER: c

The two physical principles that make rotational atherectomy possible are *differential cutting* and *orthogonal displacement of friction* (Reisman M. *Guide to Rotational Atherectomy.* Birmingham, MI: Physicians' Press; 1997:5).

Differential cutting—differences in substrate composition—allows one material to be selectively ablated while another is spared: healthy tissue has elastic properties and therefore can deflect from the cutting edges of the diamond microchips.

Orthogonal displacement of friction occurs when friction between sliding surfaces in contact is minimized by a sliding motion perpendicular to the contact surface. This allows the passage of the burr through diseased segments of the artery.

High-speed rotational atherectomy may result in the formation of microcavitations that are relatively large but collapse quickly. No deleterious effect has been described so far.

During rotablation atherectomy, there is thermal injury due to heat generation. An intermittent or oscillating technique generates the least amount of heat when applied with minimal decelerations (*J Am Coll Cardiol* 1996;27:292A).

16.   With regard to the guide catheter selection when performing a rotational atherectomy, all of the following statements are TRUE, **EXCEPT:**

    a. Significant support or deep intubation is extremely important when performing rotational atherectomy.
    b. The guide catheter inner diameter should be 0.004″ larger than the largest burr used.
    c. Guider catheters with side holes are generally recommended.
    d. Coaxial alignment is of paramount importance.

ANSWER: a

Deep intubation in order to have significant support is not generally needed with this device, since activation of the burr provides orthogonal displacement of friction, facilitating the advancement of the burr through the vessel.

Oversizing of the guider catheter is helpful because larger catheters will limit the contact between the burr and the inner surface of the guider catheter. It is recommended that the inner diameter of the guider to be 0.004″ larger than the burr. For example, a 9F catheter will accommodate up to a 2.38 mm burr.

Side holes are recommended because they provide increased perfusion and help particle clearance.

Coaxial alignment is very important in rotablation atherectomy, reducing the tension on the guidewire when advancing the burr (Reisman M. *Guide to Rotational Atherectomy*. Birmingham, MI: Physicians' Press; 1997:44).

17.   Of the following statements regarding coronary thrombus, all are FALSE, **EXCEPT:**

    a. Transluminal extraction catheter atherectomy eliminates the "no reflow" phenomenon or distal embolization.
    b. Rotablation atherectomy can be used in certain cases of coronary stenosis associated with angiographically visible thrombus.
    c. The insertion of stents in vessels with diameter <2.5 mm has been associated with increased mortality rate secondary to abrupt closure.
    d. Once coronary thrombus is present, the risk of distal embolization and no reflow is almost equal in native vessels and in vein grafts.

ANSWER: c

A mortality rate of 16% has been associated with insertion of stents in arteries with diameter smaller than 2.5 mm secondary to abrupt closure, compared to 4% in patients with larger vessels.

TEC is commonly used for thrombus extraction from vein grafts. Dissections are common and the risk of "no reflow" secondary to distal embolization is not entirely eliminated (8% to 12% of vein grafts). TEC does not reduce restenosis.

Intracoronary thrombus is a contraindication to rotablation atherectomy.

Angioplasty-related distal embolization is more frequent in vein grafts than in native vessels.

18.   Which one of the following statements regarding coronary artery perforations is TRUE?

    a.   In treating class I and II coronary perforations, reversal of heparin anticoagulation is usually sufficient.
    b.   Aspirin and heparin should be stopped in all cases of coronary perforation.
    c.   Regardless of the device used for coronary revascularization, the risk of perforation is increased when complex lesion morphology is present (angulated segment, total occlusion, bifurcation).
    d.   Balloon rupture is not associated with coronary artery perforation.

ANSWER: c

The frequency of coronary artery perforation is 1% to 2% (higher risk with excimer laser, TEC). It is more common in the elderly and in women. Regardless of the device used, the risk of coronary perforation is higher when complex lesions are treated.

Most of the time, the perforation is evident at the time of angiography, but about 10% of cases may manifest as delayed cardiac tamponade. The 4 types of coronary perforations described are:

- type I: extraluminal crater without extravasation
- type II: pericardial or myocardial blush without contrast jet extravasation
- type III: extravasation through frank perforation
- type IV: perforation into an anatomic cavity or coronary sinus

The treatment for types I and II is prolonged balloon inflation; aspirin and heparin are usually continued. In the case of more severe perforation, anticoagulation should be reversed and prolonged perfusion balloon dilatations performed in the hope that the leak will be sealed. If there is active or recurrent bleeding with hemodynamic compromise, the patient should be sent for revascularization. Thirty to forty percent of patients who develop perforation require operative intervention (*Cathet Cardiovasc Diagn* 1994;32:206–212). Stenting has been used to control the bleeding without surgery (*Cathet Cardiovasc Diagn* 1993;30:169–172). Autologous vein-coated stents have been used in rare situations (*Cathet Cardiovasc Diagn* 1996;38:175–178).

Balloon rupture is associated with increased risk of coronary artery perforation and dissection; pinhole leaks are more dangerous than longitudinal tears.

19.   Which one of the following patients is less likely to develop contrast-induced nephropathy?

    a. A 75-year-old man admitted with 4 days history of diarrhea.
    b. A 55-year-old with recent diagnosed multiple myeloma.
    c. A 39-year-old with history of cirrhosis.
    d. A 55-year-old woman with history of minimal change glomerulonephritis 20 years ago and a creatinine of 1.1 mg/dL.

ANSWER: d

The most important risk factor for the development of contrast-induced nephropathy is baseline renal dysfunction.

Contrast nephropathy is due to acute tubular necrosis. The creatinine level starts to rise in the first 24 hours, reaching a peak in 2 to 5 days. Recovery occurs in 75% of cases in 1 to 2 weeks. If the creatinine level is greater than 2.5 mg/dL prior to injection of contrast agent, more than one third of patients will have a creatinine rise ≥ 1 mg/dL. Other potential risk factors include: diabetes, age greater than 60 years, dehydration, recent exposure to large amounts of contrast media, congestive heart failure with low cardiac output, impaired hepatic function, multiple myeloma (*Cardiac Imaging: A Companion to Braunwald's Heart Disease.* Philadelphia: W.B. Saunders Co.; 1991:188). The patient with a remote history of reversible renal impairment is not at higher risk of contrast-induced nephropathy than the average population.

20.   These substances dissociate into cations and iodine-containing anions.

21.   These substances go into solutions as single neutral molecules.

22.   These substances contain calcium-chelating properties.

23.   The osmolality of these agents is 600 to 900 mOsm/kg as compared to the osmolality of human plasma of 300 mOsm/kg.

    a. Monomeric ionic contrast agents
    b. Nonionic, low-osmolality contrast agents

ANSWERS: 20-a, 21-b, 22-a, 23-b

The ionic, monomeric contrast agents dissociate into cations and iodine-containing anions, resulting in solutions with high osmolality (1940 mOsm/kg). The hypertonicity of these compounds produces sinus bradycardia, AV blocks, prolongation of QRS and QT intervals, ST depression, giant T wave inversion, decreased contractility, and increased left ventricular end-diastolic pressure. Another reason for these effects is the presence of calcium-chelating properties of some of these agents.

The nonionic, low-osmolality agents (iohexol, iopamidol) go into solution as single neutral molecules. Thus, their osmolality is reduced (<850 mOsm/kg). These agents do not contain calcium-chelating substances and therefore they have less hemodynamic and electrocardiographic effect when compared to ionic, hyperosmolar agents. Clots are more likely to form when these agents mix with blood.

Braunwald E. *Heart Disease*. Philadelphia: W.B. Saunders Co.; 1997:245.

24.   Initial frame

25.   The flow in this vessel is usually slower (on average 1.7 times)

26.   Distal landmark for the RCA

27.   Distal landmark for the LCX

28.   Distal landmark for the LAD

    a. First branch arising from the RCA after the origin of the PDA, regardless of its size
    b. Distal PDA
    c. Most distal branch of the LAD ("whale's tail")
    d. First frame in which the contrast fully enters the artery
    e. Distal AV groove circumflex
    f. Longest marginal branch beyond the lesion
    g. LAD
    h. RCA

ANSWERS: 24-d, 25-g, 26-a, 27-f, 28-c

The TIMI frame count was developed to overcome some of the subjectivity of the usual TIMI flow and to make it a continuous rather than categorical angiographic index:

Grade 0: no perfusion
Grade 1: penetration without perfusion
Grade 2: partial perfusion, the rate of entry into the vessel dis-
tal to the obstruction or its rate of clearance is per-
ceptibly slower
Grade 3: complete perfusion

The first frame used is the one in which the contrast fully enters the artery. This occurs when 3 criteria are met: 1) a column of nearly full or fully concentrated dye must extend across the entire width of the origin of the artery; 2) dye must touch both borders of the origin of the artery; and 3) there must be an antegrade motion to the dye.

The LAD flow is usually slower than the other vessels, perhaps due to its length; the correction factor is 1.7 (corrected TIMI frame count [CTFC]) and the average normal CTFC for any vessel is approximately 22 ± 2.

The biggest advantage of this count is its reproducibility and better differentiation between TIMI 2 and 3 readings. This in turn may have prognostic implications (*Circulation* 1996;93:879–888).

29.   Regarding stenting of venous graft lesions, which statement is TRUE?

    a. Balloon angioplasty of venous graft lesions has similar clinical outcome as stenting.
    b. The radial force is not important in stenting venous graft lesions, as the elastic recoil is minimal.
    c. Directional atherectomy provides similar or better efficacy than stents for vein graft disease.
    d. The outcome of the stent implantation is not dependent upon the age of the conduit.

ANSWER: d

The degeneration of SVGs begins immediately after surgery. The changes affect not only the intimal and medial layers but also the adventitia. This results in severe fibrosis and increased elastic recoil, which may require high-pressure balloon dilatation and/or lesion debulking. Restenosis after angioplasty in mature vein grafts ranges from 45% to 68% (*The Stenter's Notebook*. Birmingham: Physicians' Press; 1998:100). Stents are particularly indicated in ostial lesions in which the results are frequently not acceptable after PTCA. The rate of restenosis is significantly lower with stenting of de novo graft lesions (20%), as it was shown in observational reports (*J Am Coll Cardiol* 1995;26:704–712; *Am J Cardiol* 1994;74:1187–1191).

It must be emphasized that a recent randomized trial whose primary endpoint was the angiographic rate of restenosis after stent implantation in SVGs compared to plain PTCA showed a trend toward reduced restenosis rate with stenting versus PTCA (37% versus 46%; *P*=0.24), but statistical significance was not reached. On the other hand, the rate of clinical events (death, MI, repeat bypass surgery, revascularization of the target lesion) was significantly better for the stent group (73% versus 58%; *P*=0.03) (*N Engl J Med* 1997;337:740–747).

Because of fibrotic changes that take place in venous conduits, the radial force exerted by stents is very important in order to counteract the important elastic recoil. Removal techniques have not had a better outcome than plain angioplasty in treating venous graft lesions (*J Interven Cardiol* 1997;10:195–205). It is important to mention that the fibrotic nature of ostial lesions may require debulking techniques before the stent is implanted.

The results of stent implantation are not dependent upon the age of the graft as opposed to the results of PTCA (*J Am Coll Cardiol* 1993;21(suppl A):31A.; *J Am Coll Cardiol* 1995;26:704–712).

30.   When approaching a left IMA graft for revascularization, all of the following considerations are TRUE, **EXCEPT:**

    a.   Use of 60° LAO projection is useful when the subclavian artery is tortuous.
    b.   There is a high rate of distal embolization, associated with "no reflow."
    c.   A right Judkins catheter can be used.
    d.   Pretreatment with nitroglycerin and calcium channel blockers is indicated.

ANSWER: b

The 10-year patency of IMA grafts is 95%; despite this good long-term prognosis after surgery, stenoses may appear in the body of the graft. These lesions are amenable to revascularization. The initial success rate is high (>80%) and the rate of acute complications is low. The risk of no reflow is specific to venous grafts and may complicate 15% of cases. The restenosis rate for IMA lesions is less than 20%, and it is lower for the distal anastomotic site than it is for the body of the graft (*J Am Coll Cardiol* 1995;25:139A).

The 60° LAO projection could be very useful when difficult cannulation of the subclavian artery is encountered, because this view permits visualization of the great vessels take off. The right Judkins catheter is an alternative to the IMA guiding catheter.

Occasionally it is very difficult to engage the guiding catheter from the femoral approach; in such cases, a brachial access can be successful using an IMA or JR catheter for the ipsilateral approach and Simmons of Castillo guiders for the contralateral approach. Long shaft balloons (150 cm) or short guiding catheters (90 cm) may be required.

IMA conduit is prone to dissection and vasospasm; therefore, pretreatment with nitroglycerin and calcium channel blockers is indicated.

31. Stenting is indicated in all of the following situations, **EXCEPT:**

   a. Ulcerated lesions
   b. High eccentricity
   c. Intraluminal thrombus
   d. Total occlusion
   e. Highly calcified lesions

ANSWER: e

Rotational atherectomy is perhaps most suitable for highly calcified lesions; there is no agreement whether added stenting offers a benefit.

Most published results suggest that any device can be used for eccentric and ulcerated lesions with over 90% success rate; however, clinical experience suggests that stenting is indicated. The higher restenosis rates for total occlusions suggest that stenting is of benefit.

I.C. thrombus used to be a contraindication for stenting before the routine use of high-pressure balloon and ticlopidine; this is no longer the case and stenting is now used in the primary angioplasty setting. Also, antiplatelet therapy (abciximab) has greatly reduced acute complications in this setting.

32.   True bifurcational lesions (stenosis >50% involving the main vessel and the ostium of its side branch), can be treated with:

    a. Rotational atherectomy followed by balloon inflation
    b. Directional atherectomy followed by balloon inflation
    c. Balloon angioplasty alone
    d. Rotational atherectomy followed by stenting
    e. All of the above

ANSWER: e

Any of the above techniques can be used for treatment of bifurcation lesions, with the potential risk of side-branch occlusion due to "snow plow" effect, dissection, spasm, and thrombosis.

Debulking techniques can be used successfully to treat bifurcation lesions. The CAVEAT-I trial showed that when compared to PTCA, DCA has had higher initial success rates and less restenosis but more ischemic complications. Regarding the use of rotational atherectomy, there is a higher potential risk due to inability to protect the side branch. Stenting of the parent vessel is done successfully, with low risk of side-branch occlusion.

ELCA is not recommended in bifurcation lesions because of an increased rate of complications.

33.   The usual dose of heparin required for coronary angioplasty is:

    a. 10,000 units initially, and 1000 units every hour thereafter
    b. 70 U/kg of weight
    c. 100 U/kg of weight
    d. 15,000 units

ANSWER: c

Weight-adjusted heparinization is most adequate to achieve therapeutic anticoagulation and also to reduce bleeding complications. The target ACT is 300 to 350 seconds. If abciximab is used, then the heparin dose is lowered to 70 U/kg to achieve an ACT of 200 to 250.

The EPILOG trial showed significant reduction in ischemic complications without increase in major bleeding complications in patients receiving abciximab + weight-adjusted heparin.

The ACT range is largely empiric and is based on the prevention of fibrin deposition within the extracorporeal circuit in patients undergoing bypass surgery. Only retrospective data have been used to correlate ACT readings with complications (ie, acute vessel closure).

34.   Seventy-five percent lesion in mid LAD with 60% lesion at the ostium of second diagonal branch, which is a 2.2 mm diameter vessel originating from the LAD lesion.

35.   Eighty percent proximal LAD with a 1.5 mm diameter first diagonal branch whose ostium has a 70% stenosis.

36.   Eighty percent proximal LCX at the take off of an obtuse marginal branch which has a diameter of 2.2 mm.

37.   Ninety percent mid LAD with a 2.7 mm diameter diagonal that arises immediately beyond the lesion and is free of disease.

   a. Side-branch protection recommended
   b. Side-branch protection not recommended

ANSWERS: 34-a, 35-b, 36-a, 37-b

The majority of bifurcation lesions involve the LAD and diagonal branch.

The key problem when treating bifurcation lesions is the presence of a side branch. Side-branch protection is needed in the following situations:

• Anticipated technical difficulty passing the wire in the side branch.
• Large amount of viable myocardium supplied by the side branch (any side branch with a diameter >2.0 mm

with or without ostial disease if it takes off from the parent vessel lesion).

Risk of side-branch occlusion is low and protection is not necessary in the following situations:

- side branch with a diameter less than 1.5 mm, which would not receive a bypass graft.
- side branch that is normal and uninvolved in the parent vessel lesion but in jeopardy due to transient occlusion during inflation of the balloon.

An acutely occluded side branch can be reopened in more than 75% of cases if the ostium is free of disease but in less than 50% of cases if the ostium is significantly diseased.

There is a low risk of MI after side-branch occlusion, probably due to the phenomenon of spontaneous recanalization of the side branch.

38.   Of the following statements regarding the left lateral projection, all are TRUE, **EXCEPT:**

    a. The mid portion of the RCA can be seen well without the excessive motion of a straight RAO view.
    b. The anastomosis of left IMA (LIMA) to mid or distal LAD is seen very well in this view.
    c. Proximal and distal LAD and proximal LCX can be well visualized.
    d. The LM ostium can be frequently seen in this projection.

ANSWER: d

The best views to evaluate the *ostium* and the *proximal LM* are:

- LAO caudal
- AP projections

The *distal LM* and *LM bifurcation* can be seen well in shallow RAO caudal.

The left lateral projection offers a good radiographic penetration. This view has less motion when the mid RCA is evaluated, compared to straight RAO projection. It is the best view to evaluate the anastomosis LIMA-mid/distal LAD.

39.   RCA superior orientation ("shepherd's crook")

40.   RCA inferior orientation

41.   Tortuous LCX

    a.   Hockey stick
    b.   Extra back-up (EBU)
    c.   Multipurpose
    d.   Castillo

ANSWERS: 39-a, 40-c, 41-b

For horizontal or superior orientation of RCA take off, appropriate options are: hockey stick, Amplatz-left catheter, and Voda-right; Arani 75 can be used as well. When the vessel is very tortuous and when there is need for strong back-up, Voda and Arani are indicated (support is provided by the opposite aortic wall rather than the sinus of Valsalva).

For inferior orientation of RCA, multipurpose and Amplatz-right catheters are good options.

To engage the LCA, a Judkins catheter is usually sufficient. When there is need for increased back-up support, one of the Q-shaped guiders can be used: doctor's choice, Q, XB (extra back-up), EBU (extra back-up), or Amplatz-left (especially for inferiorly positioned LCX). When the vessel is tortuous or calcified, or if the lesion to dilate is situated distally, a guider catheter which derives support from the opposite aortic wall may be preferable.

The Castillo catheter is used for brachial approach and it has an Amplatz configuration.

42.   Good torque control

43.   Increased flexibility

44.   Kink-resistant

45.   Good support and trackability

  a. Unicore guidewires
  b. Floppy guidewires/stainless steel wires
  c. Glidewires/nitinol wires

ANSWERS: 42-a, 43-b, 44-c, 45-a

The unicore guidewires offer an excellent torque control, minimize the prolapse, and provide support and increased tracking of the balloon (heavy-duty wires).

The dual-core wires are flexible and less steerable.

The nitinol guidewires (Glidewires; Boston Scientific, Watertown, MA) are kink-resistant; because of a hydrophilic coating, they can be used in very severe or total occlusions. The Magnum wire (Schneider, Bulach, Switzerland) (1 mm olive-shaped tip) can be used as well for total, chronic occlusions.

46.   Of the following statements regarding stent deployment failure, all are TRUE, **EXCEPT:**

  a. Proximal vessel tortuosity and/or calcification are associated with increased risk of stent dislodgement.
  b. In certain circumstances, automatic power injection can be used to deploy a stent.
  c. Stent embolization, although annoying, is harmless.
  d. Occasionally, emergency CABG is necessary.

ANSWER: c

The causes of stent deployment failure are proximal vessel tortuosity and/or calcification, balloon rupture, and "watermelon seed" slippage of the balloons allowing non- or partial deployment, inadequate stent profile, and operator error.

The rare situation in which the stent-balloon ruptures before the stent is deployed can be overcome by using an automatic power injector: 50% contrast at a rate of 20 cc/s injected over 0.25 seconds (pressure limit of 200 to 400 psi) (*Cathet Cardiovasc Diagn* 1995;35:211–215).

Stent embolization is generally harmless, with the exception of cerebral embolization, which may result from stent manipulations in the ascending aorta (*Cathet Cardiovasc Diagn* 1993;30:166–168).

When stent rescue techniques (snares, loops, forceps, and bioptomes) fail and the misplaced or incompletely deployed stent is a source of mechanical total occlusion with significant clinical repercussions, emergency CABG is recommended.

47.   Stenting can safely be used in the following situations:

  a. SVGs
  b. Long lesions (>15 mm)
  c. Acute closure
  d. Prior restenosis
  e. Chronic total occlusions
  f. a, c, d
  g. a, b, c, d, e

ANSWER: g

SVGs benefit from stenting with higher technical and procedural success and less clinical events, and probably less restenosis (SAVED trial).

Acute closure is best treated with stenting, which has been shown to lower the need for emergency bypass surgery (from 3% to 5% to around 1%) as well as the restenosis rates (TASC II & STENT-BY trials).

Target vessel revascularization is reduced with stenting in restenotic lesions (REST interim analysis 12% versus 37% in favor of stenting).

Randomized trials comparing balloon angioplasty with stenting have excluded lesions greater than 15 mm in length. Lesion length was associated with increased incidence of acute complications and restenosis (up to 50%); newer reports on stenting of long lesions show a procedural success of greater than 90% and low rate of acute thrombosis (1.5%) and restenosis (35%). Some of the investigators used IVUS-guided stent deployment. The results are encouraging, although results from randomized trials are not available.

Chronic total occlusions have lower restenosis and target vessel revascularization rates when stenting is used (32% versus 74% and 22% versus 42%, respectively) (SICCO. *J Am Coll Cardiol* 1996;28[6]:1444–1451).

48.   Stenting of small vessels (<3.0 mm in diameter) reduces restenosis.

    a. True
    b. False

ANSWER: b

The early randomized trial excluded stenting in small vessels, likely due to the higher thrombosis rates present then. However, both the STRESS and Benestent 2 trials had a sizable number of small vessels in their series. Retrospective analysis of stenting of those vessels in those trials revealed no benefit.

The STRESS IV study is comparing directly these groups prospectively. Until those data are available, stenting of vessels less than 2.75 mm should be done only for bail-out indications.

49.   Multi-Link

50.   Wiktor

51.   Radius

52.   GFX

    a. Slotted-tube
    b. Mesh (self-expanding)
    c. Coil
    d. "Hybrid"

ANSWER: 49-a 50-c 51-b 52-d

Slotted tubes provide better scaffolding but are more rigid and hence less trackable through tortuous anatomy or calcified vessels. The Multi-Link (ACS, Santa Clara, CA) and its newest redesign (Duet), mounted on a high-pressure balloon, are more flexible than the older prototype. The Crown stent (Cordis, Johnson & Johnson, New Brunswick, NJ) has good radial strength, grows up to 5.5 mm, and is mounted on a high-pressure balloon; but it is more rigid. The NIR stent (Boston Scientific Scimed) also has good radial strength and flexibility.

Self-expanding stents such as the nitinol Radius stent (Scimed) have good deliverability and scaffolding.

Coil stents such as the Wiktor stent (Medtronic, Inc., Minneapolis, MN) suffer from poor axial support but have good radio-opacity. The Gianturco-Roubin (GR II; Cook, Inc., Bloomington, IN) is the only stent that has a long length (40 mm); it is very trackable but suffers from significant recoil, which probably explains its higher restenosis rates.

The Wallstent (Schneider) is a *self-expanding* stent that is very flexible, with good scaffolding. It shortens by as much as 20% (therefore it is difficult to size).

Hybrid stents such as the Micro II stent (Arterial Vascular Engineering, Santa Rosa, CA) and its enhanced model GFX stent, have a coil design joined together with flexible elements to emulate the scaffolding of a slotted tube; they are more deliverable at the expense of less radial support.

53.   Which of the following is not associated with complications during rotational atherectomy?

   a.   Decelerations >5000 rpm
   b.   Higher platform rpm
   c.   Short runs
   d.   Duration of decelerations >10 seconds

ANSWER: c

The use of short runs (15 to 30 seconds) is encouraged, as they avoid excess heat generation (known to activate platelets) and allow the microvasculature to assimilate the atherosclerotic debris. In addition, the use of vasodilators, as well as abciximab, during runs is suggested (*Circulation* 1996;94[suppl I]:I248), because it allows resolution of ST changes and angina.

The STRATAS study (*J Am Coll Cardiol* 1997;29[suppl A]:499A) revealed that decelerations increase complications.

In many laboratories, the platform speed continues to be decreased, as a way of reducing heat generation.

54.   Intracoronary administration of thrombolytics is an effective therapy for acute coronary syndromes and the presence of thrombus by angiography.

    a. True
    b. False

ANSWER: b

The incidence of adverse cardiac events and acute closure has actually increased with the use of urokinase. Therefore, this is probably of no benefit (*Circulation* 1994;90:69–77). Furthermore, the introduction of abciximab has improved the procedural success in these settings (*Lancet* 1997;349:1429–1435).

55.   Of the following statements regarding pacemaker use during rotablation atherectomy procedure, all are TRUE, **EXCEPT:**

    a. Pacemaker should be used when treating ostial LAD, ostial RCA, or ostial LCX.
    b. Temporary pacemaker is recommended when rotablation of RCA or dominant LCX is performed.
    c. Use of large burrs may be associated with AV block and therefore need for temporary pacemaker.
    d. Use of abciximab has significantly decreased the need for temporary pacemaker insertion during rotablation atherectomy.

ANSWER: d

Temporary pacemaker insertion is indicated in cases of rotational atherectomy of RCA, dominant LCX, or ostial LAD, as well as in situations where large burr use (>2.25 mm) is anticipated (Reisman M. *Guide to Rotational Atherectomy*. Birmingham, MI: Physicians' Press. 1997:41–42).

There are no data to suggest that use of abciximab should be protective against AV block during rotablation atherectomy.

56.   Of the following statements regarding excimer laser coronary atherectomy (ELCA), all are TRUE, **EXCEPT:**

    a. The excimer laser emits pulsed infrared laser light at 308 nm.
    b. Saline infusion technique has allowed a decrease in rate of acute complications related to ELCA.

    c.   Once dissection is present, the increase in laser energy can be danger-
ous.

    d.   Bifurcation lesions, highly eccentric lesions, and uncrossable total oc-
clusions are contraindications to ELCA use.

ANSWER: a

The excimer laser emits *ultraviolet light,* not infrared light. The
laser energy ablates inorganic material without generation of
heat. The laser energy is avidly absorbed when blood or contrast
dye are present, producing intimal dissection secondary to
acoustic effects. Hence, the saline infusion, following a carefully
established protocol, should be used; with this technique the rate
of dissection has been shown to be significantly reduced (*J Am
Coll Cardiol* 1995;26:1264–1269).

If dissection is present, application of additional laser energy is
contraindicated.

ELCA is contraindicated in situations where there is a serious risk
of dissection or perforation (lesions in very tortuous vessels, already dissected vessel); directional ELCA should be used for eccentric or bifurcation lesions and excimer laser guidewire for un-
crossable total occlusions.

57.   Of the following statements regarding IVUS, all are TRUE, **EXCEPT:**

    a.   It uses frequencies of 20 to 40 MHz.

    b.   Synthetic phased array devices are more flexible and have better
guidewire tracking than mechanical devices.

    c.   Optimal stent deployment criteria by IVUS includes stent symmetry
(symmetry index >0.7), absence of echo-free space between the stent
and the wall, adequate cross-sectional area (CSA) ratio of stent to reference vessel greater than 0.8, and no edge tear.

    d.   Septals and diagonal branches are indistinguishable when IVUS of the
LAD is performed.

ANSWER: d

Septal branches come out of LAD at a 90° angle, and diagonal
branches come out at a sharper angle.

For practical purposes, the optimal deployment of a stent should
show by IVUS full apposition of the struts, more than 80% resid-

ual lumen area, no edge dissections, and a symmetry index greater than 0.7 (defined as the ratio of major to minor diameters).

Newer transducers use higher frequencies, which have better image quality and less penetration.

58.   Luminal vessel detail

59.   Clot versus dissection

60.   Functional evaluation of a stenosis

61.   Diffuse disease

62.   Arterial wall and vessel dimension

    a. Doppler wire
    b. IVUS
    c. Angioscopy

ANSWERS: 58-c, 59-c, 60-a, 61-b, 62-b

I.C. angioscopy provides direct information regarding the endoluminal area, and is a superior tool for detection of thrombi (*N Engl J Med* 1992;326:287–291).

CFR determined with the Doppler wire, with use of vasodilator agents (adenosine, papaverine, dipyridamole), suggests a functionally significant stenosis if less than 2.0. If normal CFR is found, it is safe to defer the interventional procedure, with a low rate of lesion progression in the following year (*J Am Coll Cardiol* 1997;30[3]:613–620).

IVUS offers detailed information about the arterial wall and presence of diffuse disease, which may very easily be missed by angiography.

63.   Of the following statements regarding rotablation atherectomy, all are TRUE, **EXCEPT:**

    a. Rotational speed fall >5000 rpm below the platform speed allows generation of heat, large particles, and endoluminal trauma.

b. Any 0.014″ guiding wire can be used for rotablation, as long as it has a length of >300 cm.
c. The internal diameter of the guiding catheter should be 0.004″ larger than the burr diameter.
d. The rotablation burr is diamond-coated only on the leading half.

ANSWER: b

All rotablator wires are 0.009″ in diameter and 325 cm in length. There are two flexible wires (RotaWire Floppy [Scimed] is most flexible, and Standard), two stiff wires (Extrasupport, type A and type C), and one intermediate wire (RotaWire Support); the stiffer the wire, the higher the wire bias. All wires have a distal spring with a 0.014″ or 0.017″ radio-opaque tip. If the burr detaches, it can be retrieved by removing the guidewire.

Forceful advancement of the rotablator results in a drop of more than 5000 rpm from the speed platform and is associated with heat generation and vascular trauma.

The burr is diamond-coated only on the leading half.

The following burrs are available (in mm): 1.25, 1.50, 1.75, 2.0, 2.15 (accommodated by an 8F guider catheter), 2.25, 2.38 (accommodated by a large-lumen 9F guider catheter), and 2.50 (which needs a 10 F guider catheter).

64.   Of the following statements regarding "dynaglide" during rotational atherectomy, all are TRUE, **EXCEPT:**

a. It provides 50,000 to 90,000 rpm rotation when the burr is removed from the patient.
b. If the "dynaglide" light does not switch off upon deactivation of the dynaglide mode, there may be low gas pressure in the gas tank.
c. Wireclip (torque device) should be kept on the wire during "dynaglide."
d. If the vessel is small (<2.0 mm), the lesion can be crossed with "dynaglide."

ANSWER: d

"Dynaglide" is to be used ONLY for withdrawal of the burr outside the body. "Dynaglide" works on a servo control, and if resistance is met, the console will automatically deliver more air pressure to retain the predesignated speed of 60,000 rpm. Therefore, the operator will not receive the necessary feedback.

65.   Of the following statements regarding DCA, all are TRUE, **EXCEPT:**

   a. Distal cutters are available in 5F, 6F, and 7F sizes.
   b. Guiding catheters for the LCA are available in 10F and 11F, and for the RCA, 9.5F and 10F only.
   c. Small arteries (2.5 mm), moderate to heavy calcification, proximal angulation >45°, length >20 mm, extensive dissection, and degenerative SVG are all considered unfavorable for DCA.
   d. The cutter window is 10 mm and opens over a 120° arch.
   e. The balloon is attached to the opposite of the window and is designed for high-pressure inflations that will securely anchor it in position during cutting.

ANSWER: e

The balloon is designed for low-pressure inflations.

The RCA guiders are smaller, due to an increased rate of catheter-induced dissections. The most distal 2 mm is soft.

Lesions initially thought to be favorable for DCA are typically in larger vessels, proximally located and/or ostial, bifurcational (large branch) with none or mild tortuosity, and discrete.

66.   Of the following statements regarding TEC atherectomy, all are TRUE, **EXCEPT:**

   a. Any 9F guider catheter can be used as long as good alignment is obtained.
   b. The TEC guidewire can be used to cross the lesion.
   c. The cutter must be activated proximal to the lesion and advanced slowly to achieve continuous blood flow in the vacuum bottle.
   d. Dissection is frequently seen after TEC atherectomy.

ANSWER: a

The TEC is a cutting/aspiration device that uses a special guiding catheter. This is a 10F tungsten-braided guider with a soft tip. For TEC cutters ≤6.5F, a 9F guider can be used.

A special 0.014″ rigid stainless steel wire is used. The wire has a 0.021″ tip which prevents the advancement of the cutting blades beyond the guidewire. This wire can be used to cross straight forward lesions (bare wire technique is recommended); for tortuous vessels a conventional wire should be used and exchanged subsequently with the TEC wire.

The most frequently used technique is to undersize the cutter (0.5 to 0.7 cutter/artery ratio). The cutter should be activated proximal to the lesion; activating it inside the lesion results in dissection and/or distal embolization. Adjunctive PTCA can be performed for significant residual stenoses.

The procedural success is around 90% (*J Am Coll Cardiol* 1995; 25:848–854); dissection is frequently seen (≥75%) after thrombus removal using TEC atherectomy (*Am J Cardiol* 1994;74:606–609).

67.   The origin of the term LASER is:

  a.   The name of the French physicist who discovered it.
  b.   Light amplification by stimulated emission of radiation.
  c.   Light activity on atherosclerotic plaque, excision, and removal.
  d.   Light activity system/excimer radiation.

ANSWER: b

Laser energy ablates inorganic material by photochemical mechanisms (breaking molecular bonds without generation of heat). In contact with blood or contrast dye, laser energy induces an acoustic effect resulting in dissection; the use of saline infusion reduces this risk.

68.   Of the following statements regarding the excimer laser ablation, all are TRUE, **EXCEPT:**

  a.   For lesions that are noncalcified and resistant to ablation, increase *fluence* first.
  b.   For lesions that are calcified and resistant, increase *repetition rate.*
  c.   For lesions that are noncalcified and resistant to ablation, increase *repetition rate* first.
  d.   In treating resistant bypass graft lesions, increase in both *fluence* and *repetition rate* can be used.

ANSWER: c

By increasing the *fluence,* it is possible to ablate higher density tissue.

Increasing *repetition rate* results in increased cutting rate.

If resistance is still encountered, repetition rate should be increased.

For calcified lesions, increase repetition rate first.

Chapter 5

Imaging and Radiation

QUESTIONS

1. Poor fluoroscopic images are often obtained in obese patients. How would you optimize these images with regard to the x-ray control panel?

    a. Increase the focal spot and pulse width
    b. Increase the focal spot and decrease pulse width
    c. Decrease the focal spot and pulse width
    d. Decrease the focal spot and increase the pulse width

2. The clinical symptoms of acute radiation overexposure appear above what level of radiation exposure?

    a. 300 mrem
    b. 300 rem
    c. 3000 mrem
    d. 30 rem

3. The National Council on Radiation Protection (NCRP) recommended limit for annual eye dose equivalent is:

    a. 5 rem
    b. 15 rem
    c. 15 mrem
    d. 20 mrem

4. Which one of the following is NOT a way to reduce radiation exposure?

    a. Obey the "inverse square law"
    b. Select the minimum possible collimation
    c. Avoid pulsed fluoroscopy whenever possible
    d. Use cine operation with 15 instead of 30 F/s

5. What is the maximum radiation allowed by federal law for fluoroscopy at the entrance level?

    a. 10 R/min
    b. 20 R/min
    c. 50 R/min
    d. 1 R/min

6.   All of the following statements are TRUE, **EXCEPT:**

    a.   Average radiation exposure for a procedure involves a mean skin entrance dose of 32 mCi/kg of body weight (124 rads), assuming an average fluoroscopic time of 19 minutes.

    b.   The maximal occupational radiation exposure to any given operator is 5000 mem/year according to the NCRP.

    c.   Radiation exposures below 5 rem/year are considered safe for x-ray operators.

    d.   A millirem (mrem) is a unit of radiation dose. One roentgen (R) is approximately equal to 1 rem of radiation dose to tissue for most x-rays.

7.   Of the following statements regarding radiation therapy for the treatment of restenosis, all are TRUE, **EXCEPT:**

    a.   Beta radiation has a longer penetrating distance than gamma; therefore it poses a higher exposure risk for laboratory personnel.

    b.   Gamma radiation offers a higher energy but requires longer dwell times when compared with beta radiation.

    c.   A dose-response effect is observed with a "shoulder" at the lower dosages, indicating that lower doses have a very small effect on cell survival.

    d.   Continuous irradiation (ie, radioactive stents) as opposed to fractionated irradiation (or bolus) demonstrates a higher cell survival.

8.   Cataract formation in humans can be produced by a single radiation dose of:

    a.   100 rad
    b.   150 rad
    c.   200 rad
    d.   250 rad

Match the following radiation units with the corresponding definition:

9.   Roentgen (R)

10.   Rad (rad)

11.   Rem (rem)

   a. Measure of ionization delivered to a specific point.
   b. Expresses the biologic impact of a given exposure.
   c. The amount of radiation energy deposited per unit mass of tissue.

12.   Of the following statements regarding lead aprons, all are TRUE, **EXCEPT:**

   a. A $\geq$0.5 mm thickness provides approximately 88% protection at 75 kVp.
   b. Aprons should be checked for integrity with fluoroscopy every 3 years.
   c. Cracks in the lead lining result in decreased protection.

13.   All following statements are TRUE, **EXCEPT:**

   a. Radiation scatter is increased when the angle of the tube is set obliquely.
   b. Acrylic shields reduce the amount of scattered radiation.
   c. Fluoroscopy generates one fifth of the x-ray exposure of cineangiography.
   d. The source of radiation in the cardiac catheterization laboratory is the image intensifier.

14.   The radiation exposure is cumulative.

   a. True
   b. False

ANSWERS

1.   Poor fluoroscopic images are often obtained in obese patients. How would you optimize these images with regard to the x-ray control panel?

   a.   Increase the focal spot and pulse width
   b.   Increase the focal spot and decrease pulse width
   c.   Decrease the focal spot and pulse width
   d.   Decrease the focal spot and increase the pulse width

ANSWER: a

If the focus is set up at a larger size (1 mm), more x-rays will be produced, which will provide needed penetration for obese patients (the pediatric mode requires a smaller focal spot: 0.3 mm for higher resolution).

The pulse width setting can also be changed: the higher the number, the better the resolution. However, in order to maintain the maximum radiation permitted by law, the frame rate must be reduced, which in turn may create lagging of the image.

2.   The clinical symptoms of acute radiation overexposure appear above what level of radiation exposure?

   a.   300 mrem
   b.   300 rem
   c.   3000 mrem
   d.   30 rem

ANSWER: b

Acute whole body radiation exposure to:

   • less than 25 rem does not produce any observable effect
   • 25 to 50 rem produces possible blood changes but no serious injury
   • 50 to 100 rem produces blood changes and some injury

Clinical symptoms of acute radiation overexposure (>300 rem) are:

- erythema, ulceration, and blisters (1 to 3 weeks after overexposure)
- healing during the first month
- atrophy during the next few months
- after 1 year, ulceration and blistering may occur because of sun or heat burn
- amputation may be necessary after doses greater than 10,000 rem

3.   The National Council on Radiation Protection (NCRP) recommended limit for annual eye dose equivalent is:

    a.   5 rem
    b.   15 rem
    c.   15 mrem
    d.   20 mrem

ANSWER: b

NCRP recommended annual limits are:

- 5 rem = effective dose equivalent (whole body)
- 50 rem = shallow dose equivalent (skin or to each extremity)
- 15 rem = eye dose equivalent (lens of the eye)
- 0.5 rem = dose to embryo/fetus during entire pregnancy

Background and other levels are:

- 295 mrem = average background dose for U.S.
- 10 mrem = average dose from 1 chest radiograph

4.   Which one of the following is NOT a way to reduce radiation exposure?

    a.   Obey the "inverse square law"
    b.   Select the minimum possible collimation
    c.   Avoid pulsed fluoroscopy whenever possible
    d.   Use cine operation with 15 instead of 30 F/s

ANSWER: c

Pulsed fluoroscopy uses approximately 60% of the radiation that continuous fluoroscopy uses. State-of-the-art radiation systems always use pulsed fluoroscopy.

5.   What is the maximum radiation allowed by federal law for fluoroscopy at the entrance level?

    a. 10 R/min
    b. 20 R/min
    c. 50 R/min
    d. 1 R/min

ANSWER: a

This is for conventional fluoroscopy mode only. The Food and Drug Administration (FDA) limits the dose to 20 R/min in high dose rate mode. There are no established regulations for cine mode. The newer cineless labs used up to one third less radiation when compared with 35 mm movies.

6.   All of the following statements are TRUE, **EXCEPT:**

    a. Average radiation exposure for a procedure involves a mean skin entrance dose of 32 mCi/kg of body weight (124 rads), assuming an average fluoroscopic time of 19 minutes.
    b. The maximal occupational radiation exposure to any given operator is 5000 mem/year according to the NCRP.
    c. Radiation exposures below 5 rem/year are considered safe for x-ray operators.
    d. A millirem (mrem) is a unit of radiation dose. One roentgen (R) is approximately equal to 1 rem of radiation dose to tissue for most x-rays.

ANSWER: a

For fluoroscopy, the entrance or skin radiation exposure typically ranges from 1 to 2 R/min in the 9-inch mode and 2 to 5 R/min in smaller, magnified mode. For a 60-second cine run, the patient entrance or skin dose ranges from 3 to 35 rad.

7.   Of the following statements regarding radiation therapy for the treatment of restenosis, all are TRUE, **EXCEPT:**

    a. Beta radiation has a longer penetrating distance than gamma; therefore it poses a higher exposure risk for laboratory personnel.

b. Gamma radiation offers a higher energy but requires longer dwell times when compared with beta radiation.
c. A dose-response effect is observed with a "shoulder" at the lower dosages, indicating that lower doses have a very small effect on cell survival.
d. Continuous irradiation (ie, radioactive stents) as opposed to fractionated irradiation (or bolus) demonstrates a higher cell survival.

ANSWER: a

Gamma radiation has a higher penetrating power and is less densely ionizing than beta radiation. One phase 1 clinical study using this type of radiation demonstrated larger MLDs and lower mean percent stenosis as well as more favorable clinical outcomes for the patients receiving brachytherapy (*N Engl J Med* 1997;336: 1697–1703).

Beta radiation has been used in two trials. One small observational study demonstrated no benefit, whereas a second study interim analysis suggests a beneficial effect for prevention of restenosis (*Circulation* 1997:96:I219. Abstract).

8. Cataract formation in humans can be produced by a single radiation dose of:

a. 100 rad
b. 150 rad
c. 200 rad
d. 250 rad

ANSWER: c

The minimum cataractogenic dose in humans is 200 rad in a single dose. Eyeglasses made of 0.5 to 0.75 mm lead-equivalent glass should be worn by personnel exposed to radiation on a daily basis.

9. Roentgen (R)

10.   Rad (rad)

11.   Rem (rem)

a. Measure of ionization delivered to a specific point.
b. Expresses the biologic impact of a given exposure.
c. The amount of radiation energy deposited per unit mass of tissue.

ANSWERS: 9-a, 10-c, 11-b

Roentgen (R) is the measure of ionization delivered to a specific point (exposure). For example, the entrance exposure for one chest x-ray is 3 to 20 mR.

Rad (rad) represents the radiation absorbed dose. The amount of radiation absorbed per exposure depends on tissue type.

Rem (rem) is the radiation equivalent dose; it is used to describe the biologic impact of a given exposure. For x-radiation, 1 rad = 1 rem.

12.   Of the following statements regarding lead aprons, all are TRUE, **EXCEPT:**

a. A $\geq$0.5 mm thickness provides approximately 88% protection at 75 kVp.
b. Aprons should be checked for integrity with fluoroscopy every 3 years.
c. Cracks in the lead lining result in decreased protection.

ANSWER: b

Aprons should be fluoroscoped at least once a year.

13.   All following statements are TRUE, **EXCEPT:**

a. Radiation scatter is increased when the angle of the tube is set obliquely.
b. Acrylic shields reduce the amount of scattered radiation.
c. Fluoroscopy generates one fifth of the x-ray exposure of cineangiography.
d. The source of radiation in the cardiac catheterization laboratory is the image intensifier.

ANSWER: d

The source of radiation in the cardiac catheterization laboratory is the primary x-ray beam emanating from the under-table x-ray tube upward through the patient and onto the image intensifier.

A high degree of angulation increases the amount of radiation scatter.

14.   The radiation exposure is cumulative.

    a. True
    b. False

ANSWER: a

Radiation exposure is cumulative; there is no washout phenomenon.

Chapter 6

General Clinical Aspects

QUESTIONS

1. The term "angiographic-clinical dissociation," as used in the CAVEAT trial, implies:

   a. A severe coronary stenosis (>75%) does not necessarily correlate with ischemic clinical manifestations.
   b. The recommendation that a patient who received thrombolytic therapy for an acute MI should not have an angiographic study done in the 24 hours that follow.
   c. The concept of angiographic nonsignificant lesions in the setting of typical anginal symptoms.
   d. The postprocedural result does not correlate with the clinical outcome.

2. Of the following statements regarding blood transfusion after PCI, all are TRUE, **EXCEPT:**

   a. No clear source of blood loss can be identified in approximately 35% to 45% of patients.
   b. Asymptomatic patients not at risk of ischemic complications from acute anemia should receive transfusions if hemoglobin levels lower than 7 g/dL.
   c. Ambulatory care program (ACP) guidelines do not use hematocrit values as a trigger for transfusions.
   d. Age >70, procedure duration, female gender, and coronary stenting were independent predictors of blood transfusions.
   e. The risk of contracting AIDS from a blood transfusion ranges between 1:450,000 and 1:650,000.

3. Procedural success, according to the American College of Cardiology (ACC) clinical guidelines, is defined as:

   a. Achievement of anatomical success (achievement of minimal luminal stenosis diameter reduction to <50% by angiography), without major complications (death, CVA, MI).
   b. Successful relief of signs and symptoms of myocardial ischemia after the patient recovers from the procedure.

    c. Achievement of a minimal stenosis diameter reduction to <50% by angiography.

    d. Durable relief of signs and symptoms of myocardial ischemia for more than 6 months after the procedure.

4.   In patients with chronic stable angina and one vessel CAD, angioplasty is expected to accomplish all of the following, **EXCEPT:**

    a. More patients undergoing PTCA will be angina-free at 6 months compared to medically treated patients.

    b. Higher mortality for patients undergoing PTCA when compared with surgical therapy.

    c. Better than medical therapy for late (3-year) exercise capacity and hospitalizations.

    d. The same survival rate as surgery, but higher recurrent ischemic events.

5.   Of the following statements regarding revascularization for Prinzmetal angina, all are TRUE, **EXCEPT:**

    a. Coronary angioplasty appears to be an effective alternative therapy for patients with variant angina and fixed coronary stenosis.

    b. The incidence of complications related to the procedure are not more frequent than during PTCA for other types of coronary disease.

    c. The rate of restenosis is higher than in patients with fixed coronary stenosis who are undergoing PTCA.

    d. Compared to surgery for classic angina pectoris, CABG is associated with the same rate of periprocedural complications.

6.   Which one of the following patients has angiographic restenosis?

    a. A patient with diameter stenosis >50% at follow-up.

    b. A patient with residual stenosis <50% after PTCA increasing to diameter stenosis >70% at follow-up.

    c. A patient with >50% loss of the initial gain achieved after PTCA.

    d. All of the above.

7.   In humans, after angioplasty, IVUS data suggest that IH and chronic constriction contribute to what approximate percentage of late loss?

    a. 20%/80%
    b. 40%/60%
    c. 75%/25%
    d. Chronic constriction contributes ≤10% to luminal loss

8.   Of the following items, all are reasons why IMA grafting is NOT the preferred method of revascularization in patients undergoing surgery, **EXCEPT:**

    a. Radiation-induced atherosclerosis of the IMA
    b. Extensive brachiocephalic atherosclerosis
    c. Patients undergoing reoperation who have patent large-diameter atherosclerotic vein grafts, the replacement of which by the smaller caliber IMA could result in hypoperfusion
    d. Diabetic patients

9.   All of the following items represent the strongest multivariate correlates of 5-year survival after PTCA for nondiabetics, **EXCEPT:**

    a. Young age
    b. Preserved left ventricular function
    c. Absence of CHF
    d. Single vessel coronary disease
    e. Absence of hypertension

10.   All of the following items represent the strongest multivariate correlates of 5-year survival after PTCA for diabetics, **EXCEPT:**

    a. Young age
    b. Absence of CHF
    c. Female gender
    d. Single vessel disease
    e. Lack of requirement of insulin therapy

11.   The influence of diabetes mellitus on early outcome after angioplasty is best described by all of the following statements, **EXCEPT:**

    a.   Angioplasty in diabetics is associated with the same success rate as in nondiabetics.
    b.   The need for emergent CABG was the same for insulin-treated and non–insulin-requiring diabetics.
    c.   The incidence of Q wave MI and in-hospital CABG was the same for diabetics and nondiabetics.
    d.   The incidence of Q wave MI and death was the same for insulin-treated and non–insulin-requiring diabetics.

12.   Stenting of aorto-coronary SVGs is expected to achieve all of the following, when compared with balloon angioplasty, **EXCEPT:**

    a.   Larger luminal diameter immediately after the procedure.
    b.   Reduction in major cardiac events (death, MI, target vessel revascularization).
    c.   Lower angiographic restenosis rates.
    d.   Greater mean net gain in luminal diameter at 6 months.

13.   Of the following statements regarding DCA compared with balloon angioplasty, all are TRUE, **EXCEPT:**

    a.   Early randomized, prospective trials suggested a higher rate of death/MI for DCA.
    b.   Newer trials did not show this trend; however the incidence of coronary perforation and creatine kinase MB band (CK-MB) elevations was higher for DCA.
    c.   Angiographic restenosis is better for aggressive DCA.
    d.   The need for repeat revascularization is lower in the aggressive DCA group.

14.   Which of the following statements best describes the event-free survival at 5 years' follow-up post angioplasty of non-diabetics versus non–insulin-dependent diabetics versus insulin-dependent diabetics?

a. Insulin-requiring diabetics had the same long-term survival than non–insulin-requiring diabetics.
b. A difference in the survival curves between diabetics and nondiabetics becomes evident after 2 years' follow-up.
c. The difference in the survival curves between diabetics and nondiabetics attenuates in time and they parallel each other after 5 years.
d. The majority of the angioplasty procedures performed more than 1 year after the index PTCA were done at a site different from the original in nondiabetics, but at the same site in diabetic patients.

15.   Of the following statements regarding prevention of restenosis with Probucol, all are TRUE, **EXCEPT:**

a. The antioxidant effect of probucol and its lipid-lowering properties are additive in regard to decreasing restenosis after angioplasty.
b. Probucol losses its benefit when administered concomitantly with vitamins C and E and beta carotene.
c. Probucol is successful against restenosis but it is not effective against native atherosclerotic disease.
d. Probucol reduces lumen loss and restenosis rate after balloon angioplasty in small coronary arteries.

16.   Of the following statements regarding multivessel angioplasty when compared with CABG, all are TRUE, **EXCEPT:**

a. Survival and Q wave MI rates are similar at 5 years.
b. A higher number of recurrent angina and repeated revascularization procedures can be anticipated in the angioplasty group.
c. Diabetic patients have equal survival in both groups.
d. The effect of stents or minimally invasive surgery is to be determined.
e. By 5 years, two thirds of patients initially treated with PTCA would have NOT undergone surgery.

17.   Predictors of procedural success for chronic coronary occlusions include all of the following, **EXCEPT:**

    a.   Occlusion less than 3 months old
    b.   Operator's experience
    c.   No antegrade flow through the occlusion
    d.   Tapered occlusion as opposed to abrupt appearing
    e.   Absence of bridging collaterals
    f.   Occlusion less than 15 mm long and no side branches at the site of the occlusion

18.   A 75-year-old diabetic man who had a CABG 10 years ago (SVGs to LAD, RCA, and LCX) presents with recent class IV angina. His BP is 140/70 mm Hg, HR is 55 bpm on β-blockers, there are no carotid bruits, there is a (+)S4, and his distal pulses are normal. He is on maximal antianginal medication. Serum creatinine is 1.6 mg/dL. A dobutamine MIBI showed ischemia of the anterior and anterolateral walls. Coronary angiography showed mild left main disease, total occlusion of the mid LAD after a first large diagonal branch 95% proximal LCX, and total RCA. The LAD graft has a discrete 95% stenosis in the distal body of the graft, the graft to LCX is totally occluded, and the graft to RCA is patent. His ejection fraction is 50%. The patient requests to be alive and well for an important family event 3 months from now.

What recommendation would you give to this patient, taking into account all the data described above?

    a.   CABG is the therapy of choice given the multitude and the severity of this patient's coronary disease.
    b.   Multivessel PTCA is safer than CABG for this patient.
    c.   Medical treatment would be the best choice.
    d.   Only PTCA of the graft lesion is indicated.

19.   In the case presented above, which of his risk factors would not increase his perioperative morbidity and mortality?

    a.   Age
    b.   Anginal class
    c.   Diabetes mellitus
    d.   Ejection fraction
    e.   Previous CABG

20.   This patient will have a percutaneous revascularization procedure to the venous graft to the LAD. Which one of the following statements is TRUE?

    a. A 100 cm guiding catheter and a regular PTCA balloon may not work in this case.
    b. Graft age is not a predictor of distal embolization.
    c. A hockey stick guider catheter cannot be used in this case.
    d. Cardiac tamponade is a frequent complication after vein graft perforation.
    e. Stenting will not reduce the rate of clinical events.

21.   There is evidence and general agreement (class I indication) that primary PTCA is an alternative to thrombolytic therapy only in which of the following situations?

    a. PTCA is performed in a timely fashion, by cardiologists who performed more than 75 procedures per year, in a center that performs more than 200 procedures per year.
    b. PTCA is performed as a reperfusion strategy in patients who have "a risk-of-bleeding" contraindication to thrombolytics.
    c. Patients in cardiogenic shock.
    d. PTCA is performed as a reperfusion strategy in patients who fail to qualify for thrombolytics for reasons other than risk-of-bleeding contraindication.

22.   Of the following statements regarding PTCA versus CABG, all are TRUE, **EXCEPT:**

    a. Incomplete revascularization is predictive of reintervention but not survival or MI at 1 year.
    b. CABG is associated with more procedure-related MIs.
    c. Survival at 1 year is the same in both groups.
    d. PTCA in a major artery when the other vessel is occluded is contraindicated.

23.   A 50-year-old construction worker underwent PTCA and stent of a proximal 95% RCA lesion 6 months ago. He calls you to

arrange a diagnostic coronary angiography; he is very adamant about this request, which was prompted by one of his colleagues who had crescendo angina culminating with admission to the hospital last week, almost 5 months after a PTCA to RCA. Which one of the following statements is TRUE?

a. Seventy-five percent of patients with angiographic restenosis develop symptoms.
b. The stent restenosis rate is reduced by 60% compared with PTCA.
c. The prognosis of asymptomatic stent restenosis is excellent.
d. Repeat angioplasty of asymptomatic restenotic lesions is indicated to decrease the future risk of anginal symptoms.

24.   Of the following statements regarding acute MI, all are TRUE, **EXCEPT:**

a. Angioplasty is superior to thrombolytic therapy with respect to short-term mortality (30 days), nonfatal reinfarction, and intracranial bleeding.
b. Overall cost of primary angioplasty is greater than thrombolytic therapy.
c. Stenting lowers the rate of reocclusion compared to primary PTCA.
d. The rate for angiographic restenosis for stents compares favorably with angioplasty.

Answer questions 25 through 29 with TRUE (a) or FALSE (b).

25.   Ischemic complications are increased by the presence of National Heart, Lung, and Blood Institute (NHLBI) types C through F dissections.

26.   Calcific lesions are more resilient to dilating forces and are therefore more resistant to dissection.

27.   Severe dissections portend increased risk of restenosis at 6 months.

28.   The most powerful predictor of acute closure is intraprocedural appearance of complex dissection.

29.   Thrombus is more commonly detected than dissection in patients experiencing acute closure.

30.   A 68-year-old man is referred to you for percutaneous revascularization. He is asymptomatic and was found to have a 5.5 cm abdominal aortic aneurysm on a routine physical examination. His total cholesterol is 195 mg/dL; he is sedentary, does not smoke, and his father died of "heart failure" at age 81. Physical examination reveals no positive findings other than his aneurysm. A Persantine-Sestamibi stress test showed a mild anterior reversible defect in the anterior wall. He then underwent cardiac catheterization that revealed a 85% mid LAD discrete type B1 lesion after a large diagonal; the left ventricular systolic function was overall normal with mild antero-apical hypokinesis. Which of the following statements is TRUE?

   a.   Angioplasty/stent of the LAD will not make his surgery safer.
   b.   Pre- and perioperative use of β-blockers will reduce cardiac events during surgery.
   c.   Silent ischemia is as bad of a risk factor as angina.
   d.   You should tell the primary care giver that the patient needs neither abdominal surgery nor angioplasty.

31.   Regarding stenting with concomitant abciximab treatment, which of the following is TRUE?

   a.   Stenting plus abciximab reduces mortality, MI, or urgent revascularization at 30 days.
   b.   Stenting plus abciximab reduces mortality, MI, or urgent revascularization at 6 months.
   c.   Stenting plus abciximab reduces mortality at 1 year.
   d.   All of the above.

32.   A 68-year-old man is admitted to the hospital with an acute anterior wall MI. You see him in the emergency room. His

BP is 135/80 mm Hg, his HR is 85 bpm, and his physical examination is unremarkable except for an S4 gallop at the apex. LAD
is 100% occluded, RCA contains an 80% mid stenosis and ejection
fraction is 35%. He undergoes primary PTCA and is hemodynamically stable and pain free. Which one of the following statements
is TRUE regarding his outcome?

  a. The use of intra-aortic balloon pump after primary
      PTCA will reduce the infarct-related artery reocclusion.
  b. His overall clinical outcome will be improved by ad-
      junctive intra-aortic balloon pump insertion.
  c. Myocardial recovery will be hastened by the use of in-
      tra-aortic balloon pump.
  d. His outcome is not going to be influenced by the pro-
      phylactic use of the intra-aortic balloon pump.

33.   A 73-year-old woman is admitted to the hospital with a
chest pain syndrome of approximately 15 hours duration. Her
ECG reveals an evolving inferior MI. All of the following measures
are proven to improve her outcome, **EXCEPT:**

  a. Full anticoagulation with heparin
  b. Aspirin
  c. β-Blockers
  d. Cardiac catheterization and possible angioplasty

34.   Which location is less predisposed to restenosis after angioplasty of SVG lesion?

  a. Mid vein graft
  b. Distal anastomotic site
  c. Proximal anastomotic site

35.   Of the following statements regarding SVGs, all are TRUE,
EXCEPT:

  a. The native vessels should be treated whenever possible.
  b. Due to its length and flexibility, the Gianturco-Roubin
      stent is the stent of choice in treating SVGs.
  b. Multiple stent implantation is not predictive of in-
      creased risk of restenosis.
  d. TEC is associated with >10% risk of distal emboliza-
      tion and >60% restenosis rate.

36.   Which is the strongest predictor of stent thrombosis when stenting is used to treat acute MI?

    a.   The thrombus burden at the lesion site
    b.   Stent underexpansion
    c.   Low plaque mass
    d.   Use of oversized balloons

37.   Of the following statements regarding PTCA for treatment of acute MI, all are TRUE, **EXCEPT:**

    a.   The incidence of events (death, nonfatal reinfarction, and nonfatal disabling CVA) at 30 days is significantly lower in a PTCA-treated group compared to a thrombolytic group.
    b.   The rate of major events (nonfatal reinfarction, death, and target vessel revascularization) is lower in PTCA patients treated with abciximab compared to placebo.
    c.   There is no difference in outcome between patients in the PTCA group treated with heparin versus those treated with hirudin.
    d.   The ratio of TIMI 3 flow is higher after primary PTCA than after tPA.

38.   Which of the following statements regarding the presence of coronary artery thrombus are TRUE?

    a.   Angiography underestimates the presence of intravascular thrombus.
    b.   There is a clear relationship between angiographic presence of thrombus and angioplasty outcome.
    c.   Abciximab reduces the rate of adverse outcomes only in the cases when coronary thrombus is evident by angiography.
    d.   The presence of thrombus is a contraindication to stenting because of increased risk of subacute thrombosis.

Match the following to achieve the best outcome with regard to death, recurrent MI, or disabling stroke:

39.   An 80-year-old woman presents with a 2-hour history of intense chest pain, ST segment elevation in II, III, aVF, and ST segment depression in V_1 through V_2. Her past medical history is significant for chronic atrial fibrillation on warfarin therapy and a stroke 3 months ago. The physical examination shows a 50 kg elderly woman with a BP of 140/80 mm Hg and an HR of 80 bpm.

40.   A 68-year-old woman comes to the emergency room with a 3-hour history of chest pain, ST segment elevation in V_1 through V_5. Her BP is 80/60 mm Hg and her HR is 120 bpm.

41.   A 65-year-old man presents to the emergency room with a 3-hour history of chest pain (8/10); the ECG shows 3.0 mm ST depression in II, III, aVF, and V_5 through V_6; his BP is 130/70 and his HR is 78 bpm. He is started on appropriate medical therapy but 30 minutes later his chest pain and ECG changes have not resolved.

42.   A 70-year-old man presents to the emergency room with a 14-hour history of stuttering chest pain and 1 mm ST segment elevation in leads II, III, and aVF.

43.   A 35-year-old man presents to the emergency room with a 5-hour history of chest pain and ST segment elevation in leads II, III and aVF. His BP is 120/60 mm Hg and his HR is 42 bpm, in sinus with a 2:1 AV block.

    a.   Angiography and possible angioplasty emergently
    b.   Thrombolytic therapy
    c.   Either therapy
    d.   None of the above

44.   A 55-year-old man is admitted with unstable angina for the last 48 hours that is uncontrollable by medical treatment. The angiogram reveals subtotally occluded proximal LAD and faint left-to-left collaterals to the distal LAD. Which strategy is superior in reducing CK-MB leak during revascularization?

    a. Balloon angioplasty alone
    b. Stenting in addition to abciximab
    c. Stenting alone
    d. Bypass surgery

45.   Primary stenting in the setting of acute MI is associated with improved outcome.

    a. True
    b. False
    c. Unknown

46.   A 38-year-old multiparous woman presents to the hospital with a 3-hour history of chest pressure. She is 16 weeks pregnant. Her ECG shows ST segment elevation in V_1 through V_5. Her BP is 130/80 and HR is 90 bpm. Of the following statements, all are TRUE, **EXCEPT:**

    a. Her prognosis is better because she is above age 35.
    b. Catheterization is contraindicated at this time because the organogenesis is not yet completed.
    c. Her mortality ranges between 37% and 50%.
    d. Use of low-dose aspirin is safe during pregnancy.
    e. Pregnancy is a relative contraindication to thrombolytic therapy.

47.   You are performing an angioplasty of the proximal LAD in a 62-year-old male who had presented with resting angina and deep T wave inversion on the antero-septal leads on the ECG. Your visual estimation of the vessel diameter distal to the lesion is 3.25 mm, and a 3.5×15 mm stent (Crown; Cordis) is deployed at the lesion after initial balloon inflation with a 3.0 balloon with an excellent angiographic result. Which one of the following statements is TRUE?

    a. IVUS is indicated to determine stent apposition and the need for further balloon inflations.
    b. No further action is needed.
    c. The patient should not be given abciximab.
    d. Postdilate with a 3.5 mm noncompliant balloon.

48.   Patients with refractory unstable angina who are on medical therapy benefit from administration of Gp IIb/IIIa receptor antagonists.

    a. True
    b. False

Match the following:

49.   A 51-year-old male presenting with an anterior wall MI undergoes primary angioplasty with restoration in TIMI 3 flow in the vessel 2 hours after the beginning of symptoms. Left ventriculogram reveals anteroapical akinesis. ECHO performed 1 week later reveals normal left systolic function.

50.   A 55-year-old woman with class III angina undergoes a cardiac catheterization that reveals severe 3 vessel disease and ventricular systolic function with an ejection fraction of 25%. Three months after bypass surgery, she is angina-free and an ECHO reveals normal systolic function.

51.   A 53-year-old male presents 4 hours after the onset of an inferior wall MI. He reports several episodes of angina the day before that resolved each with sublingual nitroglycerin. Primary angioplasty is performed successfully and left ventriculogram reveals overall normal left ventricular function with mild inferior wall hypokinesis.

    a. Preconditioning
    b. Stunning
    c. Hibernation

52.   Of the following statements regarding the peripheral vascular complications of coronary interventions, all are TRUE, **EXCEPT:**

    a. Arteriovenous fistula may appear in 0.1% to 1.5% of cases.
    b. Retroperitoneal hemorrhage is usually due to a high femoral arterial puncture.

    c. Accurate puncture of profunda femoris artery would prevent most cases of pseudoaneurysm formation.

    d. Arteriovenous fistulae that do not close by 2 to 4 weeks should be surgically repaired.

53.   All of the following items are manifestations of cholesterol embolization syndrome, **EXCEPT:**

    a. Livedo reticularis
    b. Absent distal pulses
    c. Reduced complement level
    d. Renal failure
    e. Amaurosis fugax
    f. Abdominal pain

54.   Of the following statements regarding ELCA, all are TRUE, **EXCEPT:**

    a. Randomized trials showed similar procedural success rates and acute complication rates for PTCA and ELCA.

    b. Laser technique can be used for total occlusions that cannot be crossed with regular guiding wire and/or balloon.

    c. Presently, ELCA is not used as a "stand alone" procedure, but as an adjunctive to PTCA or stenting.

    d. At long-term follow-up there is no difference in event-free survival rate between PTCA and ELCA.

55.   A 25-year-old woman presents with initially moderate exertional dyspnea of 6 months duration. It has worsened over the last few weeks. Her physical examination reveals a II/IV late peaking systolic ejection murmur at the base—P2 was delayed. Two-dimensional ECHO reveals a 70 mm Hg systolic mean gradient across the pulmonary valve when measured by continuous wave Doppler; the infundibulum was not involved. The BEST initial treatment option is:

    a. Surgical valvotomy.

    b. Percutaneous balloon valvuloplasty with the Inoue balloon catheter (Toray Medical Co., Ltd., Tokyo, Japan).

    c. Percutaneous balloon valvotomy if there is evidence of a dysplastic valve.

    d. If the infundibulum is affected, valve replacement is preferred.

56.   Of the following statements regarding adult patients with mitral stenosis (mitral valve area ≤ 1.5 cm²), all are TRUE, **EXCEPT:**

   a. Percutaneous trans-septal mitral valvotomy is currently the initial treatment of choice for symptomatic patients.
   b. Open surgical commissurotomy is to be reserved for patients with unfavorable echocardiographic features.
   c. Restenosis after balloon valvotomy is estimated to be ~ 40% to 50%.
   d. The rate of residual atrial septal defect after balloon valvotomy is 10%.

57.   Aortic balloon valvuloplasty is recommended in all of the following clinical scenarios, **EXCEPT:**

   a. Symptomatic aortic stenosis in patients whose life expectancy is <1 to 2 years due to severe comorbid illness.
   b. Advanced age.
   c. As a "bridge" to surgery in patients whose hemodynamic instability makes them unacceptable for surgery in the present condition.
   d. Patients with moderate to severe left ventricular systolic dysfunction and a low aortic gradient and cardiac output where valvuloplasty MAY be used to determine whether the patient may benefit from valve replacement.

58.   Of the following statements regarding IMA conduit, all are TRUE, **EXCEPT:**

   a. Long-term patency of IMA grafts to vessels with <50% stenosis is lower than to vessels with more significant lesions.
   b. Perioperative anterior wall ischemia after LIMA placement is most frequently related to acute graft thrombosis secondary to artery manipulation.
   c. Long-term patency rates for LIMA to LAD are approximately 95%.
   d. The patency rate is improved if the vessel distal to the anastomotic site is free of occlusions worse than 25% of the lumen.

59.   A 49-year-old man underwent heart transplantation 3 years ago. He did well until recently, when he started to experience exertional dyspnea. A nuclear exercise stress test was positive for reversible anterior wall ischemia. Of the following statements, all are TRUE, **EXCEPT:**

     a.   Coronary disease develops by 5 years in almost half of patients.
     b.   The best way to follow up these patients would be to do annual imaging stress tests.
     c.   PTCA is not recommended in transplant patients.
     d.   A history of graft rejection and cytomegalovirus (CMV) infection increases the risk of developing coronary disease.

60.   Of the following statements concerning treatment of calcific lesions, all are TRUE, **EXCEPT:**

     a.   Rotablator atherectomy of calcific and noncalcific lesions result in equivalent procedural success rates.
     b.   The procedural success for rotational atherectomy is superior to that for PTCA of calcific lesions.
     c.   A stepped burr approach is not necessary in this particular type of lesion because of the very low risk of perforation.
     d.   Undersizing the first burr is recommended in heavily calcified lesions.

61.   Which of the following statements regarding PTCA versus medical therapy in a patient with stable angina and one vessel disease is TRUE?

     a.   PTCA will offer better survival at 6 months.
     b.   PTCA will reduce the risk of MI.
     c.   PTCA will improve this patient's exercise performance at 6 months.
     d.   PTCA will not offer any advantage over medical therapy.

62.   Your noninterventional partner sends to you a 45-year-old woman with mitral stenosis and an ECHO score of 6. She has

been in atrial fibrillation for 2 months. She has had a prior surgical commissurotomy. What should you do next?

    a.   Schedule her for catheterization and an ad hoc percutaneous mitral valvuloplasty.
    b.   Call your partner and ask if the ECHO showed right atrial thrombi and/or mitral regurgitation.
    c.   Send her back for medical treatment.
    d.   Call the surgeon to evaluate her for mitral valve replacement.

63.   Of the following statements regarding rotablator atherectomy, all are TRUE, **EXCEPT:**

    a.   The procedural success rate with rotablator atherectomy is increased by the adjunctive use of balloon angioplasty.
    b.   Restenosis rate is lower with rotablator than with angioplasty because of better debulking.
    c.   Patients with left ventricular dysfunction undergoing rotablator atherectomy may benefit from intra-aortic balloon pump insertion.
    d.   The target vessel revascularization rate may be increased by using excessive debulking.

64.   A 68-year-old man has a history of documented CAD and stable angina pectoris. He is evaluated by his cardiologist for silent ischemia with ambulatory ECG monitoring. Of the following statements regarding this patient, all are TRUE, **EXCEPT:**

    a.   If the ambulatory ECG monitoring shows episodes of nocturnal asymptomatic ischemia, this patient probably has 2- or 3-vessel disease.
    b.   The presence of silent ischemia would put this patient at a higher risk for subsequent events.
    c.   Ambulatory monitoring of myocardial ischemia is a screening test for significant CAD.
    d.   Atenolol treatment is indicated in this patient.

65.   In your opinion, revascularization for the patient described above will:

   a. Reduce the rate of hospital admissions
   b. Reduce the rate of death
   c. Reduce the rate of death or nonfatal MI
   d. All of the above

66.   Which one of the following patients would NOT benefit from carotid revascularization?

   a. A patient with amaurosis fugax and 70% to 80% carotid stenosis.
   b. An asymptomatic patient with 70% to 80% carotid stenosis.
   c. A patient with a recent transient ischemic attack and a 30% carotid stenosis.
   d. An asymptomatic patient with an absolute peak velocity of 110 cm/s at end diastole at the site of a 60% to 70% stenosis by duplex ultrasound.

67.   Of the following statements regarding the stent thrombosis, all are TRUE, **EXCEPT:**

   a. The incidence of subacute thrombosis is 0.5% to 1.0%.
   b. Acute stent thrombosis in the catheterization laboratory is associated with the highest rate of ischemic complications.
   c. Subacute thrombosis rate peaks at 3 to 5 days.
   d. The risk of stent thrombosis is lower in SVGs than in native vessels.

68.   Of the following statements regarding residual dissection after stent placement, all are TRUE, **EXCEPT:**

   a. All dissections should be covered with stents, as their presence increases the risk of subacute thrombosis.
   b. Dissections left uncovered at the end of the stent do not increase the risk of restenosis.
   c. I.C. spasm may mimic a dissection at the end of the stent.

69.   Potential revascularization options for patients who are not amenable to percutaneous or surgical means because of poor distal run-off and lack of targets include:

    a. External counterpulsation
    b. Surgical transmyocardial laser revascularization (TMR)
    c. Percutaneous TMR
    d. Angiogenesis via delivery of growth factors
    e. All of the above

70.   Of the following statements regarding TEC atherectomy, all are TRUE, **EXCEPT:**

    a. This device was designed to extract thrombi and therefore its use in SVGs eliminates the risk of distal embolization.
    b. A "dotter" effect contributes to some of the angiographic improvement after TEC atherectomy.
    c. The presence of thrombus does not influence the success rate.
    d. Calcified lesions are a contraindication to TEC atherectomy.
    e. TEC atherectomy is superior to PTCA for reducing periprocedural CK-MB elevations.

71.   Of the following statements regarding intracoronary thrombus, all are TRUE, **EXCEPT:**

    a. Rheolytic thrombectomy is a promising technique for thrombus removal.
    b. Urokinase is more effective than tPA and streptokinase for treating intracoronary thrombus.
    c. Stent thrombosis can be successfully treated with I.C. thrombolytics or Gp IIb/IIIa receptor antagonist alone.
    d. I.C. thrombolytics are useful in treating total chronic occlusions in native vessels or vein grafts.
    e. No reflow is not an indication for I.C. thrombolytics.

72.   A patient who received a 3.0 mm stent 6 months ago comes back with angina and in-stent restenosis is demonstrated. You decide to debulk the lesion using rotablation atherectomy. What would be the maximum recommendable burr size?

a. 1.5 mm
b. 1.75 mm
c. 2.0 mm
d. 2.25 mm

73.   The randomized trials of PTCA versus CABG have the following limitation(s):

a. Only a small number of patients who were suitable were randomized.
b. Long-term follow-up was limited to less than 6 years.
c. Many surgical complications were not considered in the follow-up.
d. Stents and minimally invasive surgery were not used.
e. All of the above.

74.   The question of PTCA/stent implantation versus CABG for multivessel disease is not answered as of yet.

a. True
b. False

75.   Of the following statements regarding stenting, all are TRUE, **EXCEPT:**

a. Elective stenting in de novo lesions results in less restenosis than stenting in restenotic lesions.
b. The time frame of restenosis is absolutely the same for PTCA and stent.
c. There is more intimal proliferation after stenting.
d. Poststent residual stenosis of more than 10% is associated with increased risk of restenosis.

76.   Significant subclavian artery stenosis is defined as a systolic BP difference between the two arms of:

a. 5 mm Hg
b. 10 mm Hg
c. 15 mm Hg
d. 20 mm Hg

77.   Which one of the following lesions of renal arteries is associated with higher rate of success and a lower restenosis rate?

  a. Fibromuscular dysplasia
  b. Atherosclerotic stenoses
  c. Ostial lesions
  d. Total occlusions

ANSWERS

1.   The term "angiographic-clinical dissociation," as used in the CAVEAT trial, implies:

   a. A severe coronary stenosis ($>75\%$) does not necessarily correlate with ischemic clinical manifestations.
   b. The recommendation that a patient who received thrombolytic therapy for an acute MI should not have an angiographic study done in the 24 hours that follow.
   c. The concept of angiographic nonsignificant lesions in the setting of typical anginal symptoms.
   d. The postprocedural result does not correlate with the clinical outcome.

ANSWER: d

The phenomenon of angiographic-clinical dissociation is often used in reference to the CAVEAT trials (*N Engl J Med* 1993;329: 273–274).

In the CAVEAT-I and CAVEAT-II trials, improved postprocedural results of atherectomy were associated with a poorer clinical outcome (increased rate of CPK rises and other clinical events) when compared with conventional angioplasty; therefore, the angiographic-clinical dissociation refers to the observation that better angiographic procedural results do not necessarily presage a better clinical outcome.

In the ERBAC trial, a trend toward more restenosis was observed in the rotablator and excimer laser groups (versus PTCA) despite higher rate of success before crossover and a smaller residual stenosis (*J Am Coll Cardiol* 1994;23[2]:57A). Very high ($>70\%$) restenosis rates were also reported after laser balloon angioplasty despite excellent initial lumen enlargement. A study of matched lesions also suggested that DCA may result in more IH than PTCA or stents.

2.   Of the following statements regarding blood transfusion after PCI, all are TRUE, **EXCEPT:**

   a. No clear source of blood loss can be identified in approximately 35% to 45% of patients.
   b. Asymptomatic patients not at risk of ischemic complications from acute anemia should receive transfusions if hemoglobin levels lower than 7 g/dL.

   c. ACP guidelines do not use hematocrit values as a trigger for transfusions.
   d. Age >70, procedure duration, female gender, and coronary stenting were independent predictors of blood transfusions.
   e. The risk of contracting AIDS from a blood transfusion ranges between 1:450,000 and 1:650,000.

ANSWER: b

The ACP guidelines state that crystalloid solutions should be attempted first, that a single unit of blood may be sufficient, and that asymptomatic patients not at risk of ischemic complications from acute anemia should not receive transfusions even at hemoglobin levels lower than 7 g/dL. The ACP guidelines do not use hematocrit values as a trigger for transfusion.

Age greater than 70 years, female gender, procedure duration, postprocedural use of heparin, stent implantation (pre-ticlopidine and high-pressure stent dilatation), acute MI, and intra-aortic balloon pump placement were all independent predictors of blood transfusion.

It has been estimated that the risk of contracting AIDS from a blood transfusion ranges between 1:450,000 and 1:650,000. The risk of blood-borne CMV infection, hepatitis C, or hepatitis B is as high as 1:5, 3:10,000, and 1:500,000 respectively.

Among the internal medicine subspecialties reviewed in one study, the cardiology service had the most frequent inappropriate red blood cell use (71%) (*Am J Cardiol* 1998;81:702–707).

3.   Procedural success, according to the American College of Cardiology (ACC) clinical guidelines, is defined as:

   a. Achievement of anatomical success (achievement of minimal luminal stenosis diameter reduction to <50% by angiography), without major complications (death, CVA, MI).
   b. Successful relief of signs and symptoms of myocardial ischemia after the patient recovers from the procedure.
   c. Achievement of a minimal stenosis diameter reduction to <50% by angiography.
   d. Durable relief of signs and symptoms of myocardial ischemia for more than 6 months after the procedure.

ANSWER: a

The ACC guidelines define item **a** as procedural success, item **b** as short-term clinical success, item **c** as anatomical success, and item **d** as long-term clinical success (*J Am Coll Cardiol* 1998; 31:729).

4.   In patients with chronic stable angina and one vessel CAD, angioplasty is expected to accomplish all of the following, **EXCEPT:**

   a.   More patients undergoing PTCA will be angina-free at 6 months compared to medically treated patients.
   b.   Higher mortality for patients undergoing PTCA when compared with surgical therapy.
   c.   Better than medical therapy for late (3-year) exercise capacity and hospitalizations.
   d.   The same survival rate as surgery, but higher recurrent ischemic events.

ANSWER: b

The only prospective study performed in patients with stable angina, including those with LAD and non-LAD disease (ACME Trial. *N Engl J Med* 1992;326:10), was performed in the pre-stent era. The success rate was low for today's standards (82%).

Ten percent of medically treated patients crossed over to PTCA, and 15% of angioplastied patients required a second PTCA. At 6 months, 64% of the PTCA group and 46% of the medical group were angina-free. Long-term follow-up (3 years) revealed better exercise capacity and fewer subsequent catheterizations, interventions, and hospitalizations in the PTCA group (*Circulation* 1995;92:I725).

Severe proximal LAD disease is perhaps better treated with a surgical approach. In MASS (Medical therapy, Angioplasty, or Surgery Study) the 3-year survival was similar for all 3 groups, but patients randomized to LIMA graft had significantly better event-free survival. It must be mentioned that stenting was not available (*J Am Coll Cardiol* 1995;26:1600–1605).

The treatment, however, must be individualized; factors tending to favor PTCA are younger age, cerebrovascular disease, severe chronic obstructive pulmonary disease (COPD), illness limiting survival, type A lesion, and patient desire to avoid CABG and acceptance of risks of repeat procedures. If PTCA is chosen, stenting may be indicated to reduce subsequent target vessel revascularization *(N Engl J Med* 1997;336:817–822).

5.   Of the following statements regarding revascularization for Prinzmetal angina, all are TRUE, **EXCEPT:**

    a. Coronary angioplasty appears to be an effective alternative therapy for patients with variant angina and fixed coronary stenosis.
    b. The incidence of complications related to the procedure are not more frequent than during PTCA for other types of coronary disease.
    c. The rate of restenosis is higher than in patients with fixed coronary stenosis who are undergoing PTCA.
    d. Compared to surgery for classic angina pectoris, CABG is associated with the same rate of periprocedural complications.

ANSWER: d

Compared to classic angina pectoris, coronary bypass for variant angina is associated with a higher operative risk, a higher post-operative MI rate, early graft closure, and more recurrent angina (*Chest* 1974;66:614–621).

A high technical success rate can be achieved with PTCA and the incidence of complications, including PTCA-induced coronary artery spasm, is not higher than in other patients who undergo coronary angioplasty.

The rate of restenosis is much higher (approximately 50%) in patients with variant angina than in patients with a fixed coronary obstruction, and seems to be reduced by calcium channel blockers. Small observational studies suggest an advantage to stenting (*Circulation* 1996;94:I-454).

6.   Which one of the following patients has angiographic restenosis?

    a. A patient with diameter stenosis >50% at follow-up.
    b. A patient with residual stenosis <50% after PTCA increasing to diameter stenosis >70% at follow-up.
    c. A patient with >50% loss of the initial gain achieved after PTCA.
    d. All of the above.

ANSWER: d

Angiographic restenosis has been defined in many ways.

Some definitions view restenosis as a dichotomous event (ie, either present or absent).

The most common definition of restenosis is diameter stenosis greater than 50% at follow-up (*Am J Cardiol* 1987;60:39B–43B).

The most recent NHLBI (IV) definition of angiographic restenosis is a greater than 50% loss of the initial gain achieved after PTCA.

Another way to present restenosis is to see it as an event that occurs to a variable extent in virtually all lesions. Changes in lumen diameter follow a Gaussian distribution. Cumulative distribution curves allow more effective comparisons between different interventions.

7.   In humans, after angioplasty, IVUS data suggest that IH and chronic constriction contribute to what approximate percentage of late loss?

    a. 20%/80%
    b. 40%/60%
    c. 75%/25%
    d. Chronic constriction contributes ≤10% to luminal loss

ANSWER: b

Mintz et al (*Circulation* 1993;88[suppl I]:I-654), using IVUS, showed that remodeling accounts for 60% of late luminal loss; the rest is due to IH.

The magnitude of remodeling versus IH did not vary among devices (PTCA, ROTO, DCA, excimer laser angioplasty), adjunctive PTCA, or arterial expansion during the initial procedure. On the other hand, IH is the most important process involved in stent restenosis.

8.   Of the following items, all are reasons why IMA grafting is NOT the preferred method of revascularization in patients undergoing surgery, **EXCEPT:**

    a. Radiation-induced atherosclerosis of the IMA
    b. Extensive brachiocephalic atherosclerosis
    c. Patients undergoing reoperation who have patent large-diameter atherosclerotic vein grafts, the replacement of which by the smaller caliber IMA could result in hypoperfusion
    d. Diabetic patients

ANSWER: d

IMA grafts have 10-year patency rates above 90%; they are associated with survival benefits. Diabetes is not an exclusion (*N Engl J Med* 1996;334:263–265).

9.   All of the following items represent the strongest multivariate correlates of 5-year survival after PTCA for nondiabetics, **EXCEPT:**

    a.   Young age
    b.   Preserved left ventricular function
    c.   Absence of CHF
    d.   Single vessel coronary disease
    e.   Absence of hypertension

ANSWER: e

Hypertension, although a risk factor for CAD, does not correlate with 5-year survival after PTCA. The strongest multivariate correlates of 5-year survival are, in order of importance: young age, preserved left ventricular function, absence of CHF, and absence of multivessel disease (*Circulation* 1995;91:979–989).

10.   All of the following items represent the strongest multivariate correlates of 5-year survival after PTCA for diabetics, **EXCEPT:**

    a.   Young age
    b.   Absence of CHF
    c.   Female gender
    d.   Single vessel disease
    e.   Lack of requirement of insulin therapy

ANSWER: c

The strongest multivariate correlates of 5-year survival for diabetic patients were the same as for the overall population. In addition, the lack of requirement of insulin therapy correlated independently with survival. Female sex and history of MI were marginal correlates of decreased survival (*Circulation* 1995;91: 979–989).

11.   The influence of diabetes mellitus on early outcome after angioplasty is best described by all of the following statements, **EXCEPT:**

a. Angioplasty in diabetics is associated with the same success rate as in nondiabetics.
b. The need for emergent CABG was the same for insulin-treated and non-insulin-requiring diabetics.
c. The incidence of Q wave MI and in-hospital CABG was the same for diabetics and nondiabetics.
d. The incidence of Q wave MI and death was the same for insulin-treated and non-insulin-requiring diabetics.

ANSWER: d

The success rate, the incidence of Q wave MI, and the need for CABG were the same in diabetic and nondiabetic patients.

Patients requiring insulin are generally younger, are more often females, and have worse baseline left ventricular and renal functions, higher prevalence of unstable angina, previous MI, and CHF. Despite these baseline differences, procedural and clinical successes were similar (angiographic success of 89%) as was the incidence of in-hospital major complications (3%) and the need for CABG (2.3%).

However, the Q wave MI and death were 3 times more frequent in patients requiring insulin (*Circulation* 1995;91:979–989).

12. Stenting of aorto-coronary SVGs is expected to achieve all of the following, when compared with balloon angioplasty, **EXCEPT:**

a. Larger luminal diameter immediately after the procedure.
b. Reduction in major cardiac events (death, MI, target vessel revascularization).
c. Lower angiographic restenosis rates.
d. Greater mean net gain in luminal diameter at 6 months.

ANSWER: c

Earlier observational studies suggested a restenosis benefit for stenting vein grafts; however the restenosis rate between Palmaz-Schatz and balloon angioplasty in the only prospective, randomized study was 37% and 46%, respectively, in this 220-patient trial (*P*=0.24). Despite this, the clinical and other angiographic outcomes were better for the stent group, except for bleeding complications that were probably due to the old protocol before the era of high-pressure inflations and ticlopidine/aspirin (*N Engl J Med* 1997; 337:740–747).

13.   Of the following statements regarding DCA compared with balloon angioplasty, all are TRUE, **EXCEPT:**

    a. Early randomized, prospective trials suggested a higher rate of death/MI for DCA.
    b. Newer trials did not show this trend; however the incidence of coronary perforation and creatine kinase MB band (CK-MB) elevations was higher for DCA.
    c. Angiographic restenosis is better for aggressive DCA.
    d. The need for repeat revascularization is lower in the aggressive DCA group.

ANSWER: d

The initial trials of DCA (CAVEAT and CCAT) did not involve aggressive removal of tissue or adjunctive balloon inflation. With a more aggressive approach (BOAT), a higher procedural success rate and lower angiographic restenosis rate without differences in mortality was achieved with DCA; however, the need for repeat revascularization was not changed. Primary stenting was not part of the protocol (*Circulation* 1998;97:309–311).

14.   Which of the following statements best describes the event-free survival at 5 years' follow-up post angioplasty of nondiabetics versus non-insulin-dependent diabetics versus insulin-dependent diabetics?

    a. Insulin-requiring diabetics had the same long-term survival than non-insulin-requiring diabetics.
    b. A difference in the survival curves between diabetics and nondiabetics becomes evident after 2 years' follow-up.
    c. The difference in the survival curves between diabetics and nondiabetics attenuates in time and they parallel each other after 5 years.
    d. The majority of the angioplasty procedures performed more than 1 year after the index PTCA were done at a site different from the original in nondiabetics, but at the same site in diabetic patients.

ANSWER: b

A study of 9300 nondiabetic patients and 1133 diabetics (*Circulation* 1995;91:979–989) showed the following results:

• 5-year survival was 93% in nondiabetics and 89% in diabetics (*P*<0.0001);
• the need for CABG is higher in diabetics (14% versus 23%; *P*<0.0001);

- at the end of 5 years, 43% of diabetics required repeat PTCA versus 32% of nondiabetics (*P*<0.0001);
- the difference in survival curves and the need for CABG was apparent after 2 years, and the curves continue to diverge;
- two thirds to three quarters of angioplasty procedures performed more than 1 year after index PTCA were done at a different site in all patients.

15.   Of the following statements regarding prevention of restenosis with Probucol, all are TRUE, **EXCEPT:**

   a. The antioxidant effect of probucol and its lipid-lowering properties are additive in regard to decreasing restenosis after angioplasty.
   b. Probucol losses its benefit when administered concomitantly with vitamins C and E and beta carotene.
   c. Probucol is successful against restenosis but it is not effective against native atherosclerotic disease.
   d. Probucol reduces lumen loss and restenosis rate after balloon angioplasty in small coronary arteries.

ANSWER: a

The antioxidant effect of probucol may prevent endothelial dysfunction and LDL oxidation, and in turn, modify neointimal formation and vascular remodeling involved in restenosis. The weak lipid-lowering effects of probucol cannot account for its antistenotic effect, especially in light of the fact that, in one large clinical trial, the more potent lovastatin failed to prevent restenosis (*N Engl J Med* 1994;331:1331–1337).

Probucol losses its benefit when administered concomitantly with vitamins C and E and beta carotene. Differences in lipid solubility may be responsible.

The Probucol Regression Swedish Trial reported no regression in femoral artery arteriosclerosis in patients treated with probucol. This result could be secondary to the decrease in HDL levels induced by probucol. It is possible that the drug exercises its effect when present at the time of injury (balloon angioplasty) but not when injury preexisted (established atherosclerosis).

Restenosis rate is higher after PTCA of small vessels with diameter less than 2.9 mm (M-HEART study) (*J Am Coll Cardiol*

1991;18:647–656). There are presently no clear data on the use of stents in small arteries. Clinical studies showed that probucol reduces restenosis in small vessels (mean vessel reference diameter of 2.49 mm) to 21.7% per patient (*N Engl J Med* 1997;337: 365–372). In the PART study (*J Am Coll Cardiol* 1997;29:418A), the restenosis rate in arteries smaller than 2.7 mm was 24% in the probucol group compared to 75% in the control group.

16.   Of the following statements regarding multivessel angioplasty when compared with CABG, all are TRUE, **EXCEPT:**

    a. Survival and Q wave MI rates are similar at 5 years.
    b. A higher number of recurrent angina and repeated revascularization procedures can be anticipated in the angioplasty group.
    c. Diabetic patients have equal survival in both groups.
    d. The effect of stents or minimally invasive surgery is to be determined.
    e. By 5 years, two thirds of patients initially treated with PTCA would have NOT undergone surgery.

ANSWER: c

Although it was not a prespecified group in the BARI and EAST studies, subgroup analysis seems to confer a survival advantage to surgery for diabetic patients (*N Engl J Med* 1996;335:275–276).

17.   Predictors of procedural success for chronic coronary occlusions include all of the following, **EXCEPT:**

    a. Occlusion less than 3 months old
    b. Operator's experience
    c. No antegrade flow through the occlusion
    d. Tapered occlusion as opposed to abrupt appearing
    e. Absence of bridging collaterals
    f. Occlusion less than 15 mm long and no side branches at the site of the occlusion

ANSWER: c

Presence of antegrade flow is associated with higher success rates (76%) compared to vessels with TIMI 0 flow (58%).

Successful recanalization is achieved in ~65% of attempts; however, cases were highly selected based on clinical and angiographic features that predict success. Inability to cross the stenosis with a guidewire is the most common cause of failure. Restenosis can be expected in greater than 50% of cases even after successful recanalization (*J Am Coll Cardiol* 1995;26:1–11).

18.   A 75-year-old diabetic man who had a CABG 10 years ago (SVGs to LAD, RCA, and LCX) presents with recent class IV angina. His BP is 140/70 mm Hg, HR is 55 bpm on β-blockers, there are no carotid bruits, there is a (+)S4, and his distal pulses are normal. He is on maximal antianginal medication. Serum creatinine is 1.6 mg/dL. A dobutamine MIBI showed ischemia of the anterior and anterolateral walls. Coronary angiography showed mild left main disease, total occlusion of the mid LAD after a first large diagonal branch, 95% proximal LCX, and total RCA. The LAD graft has a discrete 95% stenosis in the distal body of the graft, the graft to LCX is totally occluded, and the graft to RCA is patent. His ejection fraction is 50%. The patient requests to be alive and well for an important family event 3 months from now.

What recommendation would you give to this patient, taking into account all the data described above?

   a.   CABG is the therapy of choice given the multitude and the severity of this patient's coronary disease.
   b.   Multivessel PTCA is safer than CABG for this patient.
   c.   Medical treatment would be the best choice.
   d.   Only PTCA of the graft lesion is indicated.

ANSWER: b

The relative risks and benefits of PTCA and re-CABG in patients with previous coronary bypasses was evaluated in a nonrandomized series of patients (*J Am Coll Cardiol* 1996;28:1140–1146). Major in-hospital complications occurred more frequently in the re-CABG group. In-hospital mortality was higher in the re-CABG group compared to the PTCA group (7.3% versus 0.3%; $P<0.0001$). Q wave MI was also significantly more frequent in the re-CABG group (6.1% versus 0.9%; $P<0.0001$). Fifty percent of deaths in the re-CABG group occurred in the OR or within 24 hours of the procedure, associated with inadequate restoration of myocardial function despite maximal mechanical and pharmacologic support and technically successful procedure. In the PTCA group the early deaths were associated with grafts age greater than 12.5 years, and to dilatation attempt of unprotected LM. During the follow-up period, the overall event-free (death or MI) survival rates were similar in the PTCA and re-CABG groups. Angina class was similar in both groups at 4 years. Patients in the PTCA group required more procedures than did patients in the re-CABG group to achieve equivalent symptom relief.

Arguably, the most suitable approach to this patient is multivessel angioplasty. This will offer him the lowest in-hospital morbidity and mortality. His creatinine is of obvious concern, but this problem can be overcome by preprocedural hydration to ensure euvolemia, perform first the culprit vessel PTCA, and stage the remaining stenoses. In the case of this particular patient, the nuclear imaging study showed extensive antero-lateral ischemia, indicating the need for revascularization of the venous graft to LAD and of the proximal native LCX.

19.   In the case presented above, which of his risk factors would not increase his perioperative morbidity and mortality?

    a. Age
    b. Anginal class
    c. Diabetes mellitus
    d. Ejection fraction
    e. Previous CABG

ANSWER: d

The accepted risk factors for increased morbidity and mortality perioperatively are LM disease, anginal class III–IV, age greater than 60 years, diabetes mellitus, ejection fraction less than 40%, and incomplete revascularization (*J Thorac Cardiovasc Surg* 1987; 93:847–859).

20.   This patient will have a percutaneous revascularization procedure to the venous graft to the LAD. Which one of the following statements is TRUE?

    a. A 100 cm guiding catheter and a regular PTCA balloon may not work in this case.
    b. Graft age is not a predictor of distal embolization.
    c. A hockey stick guider catheter cannot be used in this case.
    d. Cardiac tamponade is a frequent complication after vein graft perforation.
    e. Stenting will not reduce the rate of clinical events.

ANSWER: a

For lesions involving the distal body of the graft, distal anastomosis, or native vessel beyond the anastomosis, short (90 cm) guiding catheters and/or PTCA balloon catheters with long shafts (140 to 150 cm) may be useful to reach the lesion.

Independent predictors of distal embolization include diffuse degeneration and large plaque volume, which are more frequently seen in old grafts (*Am J Cardiol* 1993;72:514–517).

A hockey stick guider catheter is a good choice for venous grafts to the LAD, since they often have a superior orientation.

Cardiac tamponade is unusual after vein graft perforation due to extra pericardial course of vein grafts and postpericardiotomy fibrosis.

A randomized trial demonstrated that using Palmaz-Schatz stents did reduce the rate of major cardiac clinical events compared to PTCA in vein grafts (*N Engl J Med* 1997;337:740–747).

21.   There is evidence and general agreement (class I indication) that primary PTCA is an alternative to thrombolytic therapy only in which of the following situations?

    a. PTCA is performed in a timely fashion, by cardiologists who performed more than 75 procedures per year, in a center that performs more than 200 procedures per year.
    b. PTCA is performed as a reperfusion strategy in patients who have "a risk-of-bleeding" contraindication to thrombolytics.
    c. Patients in cardiogenic shock.
    d. PTCA is performed as a reperfusion strategy in patients who fail to qualify for thrombolytics for reasons other than risk-of-bleeding contraindication.

ANSWER: a

In November of 1996, the American College of Cardiology and the American Heart Association published the *American College of Cardiology-American Heart Association Guidelines for the Management of Patients with Acute Myocardial Infarction.*

Only answer **a** represents a class I indication (condition for which there is evidence for and/or general agreement that a given procedure or treatment is beneficial, useful, and effective).

Answers **b** and **c** represent class IIa indications (conditions for which weight of evidence/opinion, is in favor of usefulness/efficacy of a procedure).

Finally, answer **d** belongs to a class IIb indication (usefulness/efficacy is less well established by evidence/opinion).

22.   Of the following statements regarding PTCA versus CABG, all are TRUE, **EXCEPT:**

　　　a.　Incomplete revascularization is predictive of reintervention but not survival or MI at 1 year.
　　　b.　CABG is associated with more procedure-related MIs.
　　　c.　Survival at 1 year is the same in both groups.
　　　d.　PTCA in a major artery when the other vessel is occluded is contraindicated.

ANSWER: c

In the GABI trial (*N Engl J Med* 1994;331:1037–1043) and in EAST trial (*N Engl J Med* 1994;331:1044–1050), the coronary artery bypass surgery was associated with more procedure-related Q wave MIs (8.1 versus 2.3 and 3.0 versus 0.3, respectively).

In the ERACI trial (*J Am Coll Cardiol* 1993;22:1060–1067) there was no difference in 1-year outcome between CABG patients who had all stenoses greater than 50% bypassed (complete anatomical revascularization) and PTCA patients who had revascularized only those lesions that caused ischemia (complete functional revascularization); 95% of patients were asymptomatic at follow-up. In the CABRI study (*Lancet* 1995;346:1179–1184) incomplete revascularization was predictive of reintervention, but not survival or MI at 1 year.

Several studies have evaluated the results of PTCA in a major artery when the other vessel is occluded (*J Am Coll Cardiol* 1993;22:1298–1303; *Am Heart J* 1991;122:415). The success and complication rate are acceptable. Nevertheless, many interventionalists refer such patients for CABG, particularly when the occluded vessel supplies a large myocardial territory, when left ventricular function is poor, or when target lesion has high-risk morphology for MI (eg, angulation, thrombus present, long lesion). These patients should understand that although PTCA may be a viable alternative to CABG, repeat revascularization (including CABG) may be required 30% to 40% of the time.

The RITA trial (*Lancet* 1994;344:927–930), the ERACI trial, the GABI trial, the EAST trial, and the CABRI trial showed similar survival at 1 year in the two regimen groups (CABG versus multi-vessel PTCA).

23.   A 50-year-old construction worker underwent PTCA and stent of a proximal 95% RCA lesion 6 months ago. He calls you to arrange a diagnostic coronary angiography; he is very adamant about this request, which was prompted by one of his colleagues who had crescendo angina culminating with admission to the hospital last week, almost 5 months after a PTCA to RCA. Which one of the following statements is TRUE?

    a. Seventy-five percent of patients with angiographic restenosis develop symptoms.
    b. The stent restenosis rate is reduced by 60% compared with PTCA.
    c. The prognosis of asymptomatic stent restenosis is excellent.
    d. Repeat angioplasty of asymptomatic restenotic lesions is indicated to decrease the future risk of anginal symptoms.

ANSWER: c

The prognosis of asymptomatic stent restenosis is excellent and medical treatment of these patients is appropriate.

Only 50% of those patients with angiographic restenosis develop symptoms, resulting in a reintervention rate after stenting of approximately 10% across many trials. There may be remodeling or contraction of neointimal matrix within restenosed stents allowing a late resorption of the restenotic lesion between 6 months and 3 years.

Repeat angioplasty of asymptomatic restenotic lesions before there is time for late remodeling could result in unnecessary procedures to treat angiographic restenosis, with questionable benefit.

In our specific case, you should reassure your patient and not encourage him to have the angiography as long as he is symptom-free.

24.   Of the following statements regarding acute MI, all are TRUE, **EXCEPT:**

    a. Angioplasty is superior to thrombolytic therapy with respect to short-term mortality (30 days), nonfatal reinfarction, and intracranial bleeding.
    b. Overall cost of primary angioplasty is greater than thrombolytic therapy.
    c. Stenting lowers the rate of reocclusion compared to primary PTCA.
    d. The rate for angiographic restenosis for stents compares favorably with angioplasty.

ANSWER: b

Trials of balloon angioplasty versus thrombolysis for acute MI have shown angioplasty to be superior with respect to mortality or nonfatal MI. (*N Engl J Med* 1993;328:673–679; *N Engl J Med* 1997;336:1621–1628).

The cost of primary angioplasty has been shown to be similar to or less than that of thrombolysis (*J Am Coll Cardiol* 1997;26: 901–907; *N Engl J Med* 1993;328:685–691; *Am J Cardiol* 1995;76: 830; *J Am Coll Cardiol* 1995;25[suppl]:385–415).

The rate of angiographic restenosis for nearly 600 patients who had angiographic follow-up was 23% (using the definition of >50% stenosis), comparing favorably with balloon angioplasty. The overall mortality was 6.6% with angioplasty but only 0.6% with stenting. A study from Japan showed a combined event rate (death, nonfatal reinfarction, repeat revascularization) was 38% in the balloon, but only 11% in the stent-assigned patients (*J Am Coll Cardiol* 1997;29[suppl A]:390A). The largest randomized trial reported to date (Stent PAMI) found a lower rate of restenosis with stenting compared to primary PTCA (20.3% versus 33.5%; $P<0.001$) (*J Am Coll Cardiol* 1999;33:397A). The rate of reocclusion at 6 months was also reduced in the stent group (5% versus 9%; $P=0.04$).

25.   Ischemic complications are increased by the presence of National Heart, Lung, and Blood Institute (NHLBI) types C through F dissections.

26.   Calcific lesions are more resilient to dilating forces and are therefore more resistant to dissection.

27.   Severe dissections portend increased risk of restenosis at 6 months.

28.   The most powerful predictor of acute closure is intraprocedural appearance of complex dissection.

29.   Thrombus is more commonly detected than dissection in patients experiencing acute closure.

ANSWERS: 25-a, 26-b, 27-b, 28-a, 29-b

The presence of complex dissection (types C through F) was associated with lower procedural success (75% versus 92%) and more frequent in-hospital ischemic complications (15% versus 3%) (STRESS trial). (*N Engl J Med* 1994;331:496–501).

The major risk factors of acute ischemic complications in the setting of coronary dissection after PTCA are dissection length greater than 15 mm, NHLBI dissection types C through F, residual diameter stenosis greater than 30%, residual CSA less than 2 mm², transient in-lab occlusion, unstable angina, and chronic total occlusion (*Circulation* 1991;84:II-130).

Angiographic predictors of PTCA-induced dissection are diffuse disease and angulation, as well as the following lesions: calcified, eccentric, long, and types B or C (*Am Heart J* 1993;126:39–47).

Observational studies showed that dissections occur at the junction of segments with differing elastic properties (ie, junction between calcified and noncalcified plaque), resulting in nonuniform transmission of dilating forces (*Circulation* 1992;86:64–70).

Dissection does not have impact on restenosis. Four to sixteen percent of dissections disappear in 24 hours and 63% to 93% disappear in 3 to 6 months (*J Am Coll Cardiol* 1995;25:345A; *J Am Coll Cardiol* 1995;25:139A).

The most important predictor of acute closure is the presence of severe dissection. There is a 6.5-fold increase in the risk of major complications when intimal dissection is present (10.5% versus 1.6%) (*J Am Coll Cardiol* 1992;20:701–706).

Dissection detected by angiography and angioscopy is more commonly present than thrombus in patients experiencing abrupt vessel closure (*J Am Coll Cardiol* 1992;19:926; *J Am Coll Cardiol* 1995; 25:1681; *Circulation* 1995;92:311).

30.   A 68-year-old man is referred to you for percutaneous revascularization. He is asymptomatic and was found to have a 5.5 cm abdominal aortic aneurysm on a routine physical examination. His total cholesterol is 195 mg/dL; he is sedentary, does not smoke, and his father died of "heart failure" at age 81. Physical examination reveals no positive findings other than his aneurysm. A Persantine-Sestamibi stress test showed a mild anterior reversible defect in the anterior wall. He then underwent cardiac catheterization that revealed a 85% mid LAD discrete type B1 lesion after a large diagonal; the left ventricular systolic function was overall normal with mild antero-apical hypokinesis. Which of the following statements is TRUE?

    a. Angioplasty/stent of the LAD will not make his surgery safer.
    b. Pre- and perioperative use of β-blockers will reduce cardiac events during surgery.
    c. Silent ischemia is as bad of a risk factor as angina.
    d. You should tell the primary care giver that the patient needs neither abdominal surgery nor angioplasty.

ANSWER: b

β-Blockers have been shown to reduce mortality and cardiac events in patients at moderate risk for coronary disease (*N Engl J Med* 1996;335:1713–1720).

The issue or revascularization before elective surgery is controversial and is based on only retrospective data with studies in favor of surgical revascularization (*Cardiovasc Surg* 1993; 1:552–557) or percutaneous revascularization (*Mayo Clin Proc* 1992;67:15–21).

The American College of Physicians recommends that consideration for PTCA be guided by the evidence available in the NONOPERATIVE setting (*Ann Intern Med* 1997;127:313–328); in this particular case, the issue of silent ischemia and the role of PTCA is still evolving, but given the lack of more extensive disease, mild ischemic nuclear defect, and normal left ventricular systolic function, the overall prognosis is good and is unlikely to improve a great amount after revascularization.

31.   Regarding stenting with concomitant abciximab treatment, which of the following is TRUE?

    a. Stenting plus abciximab reduces mortality, MI, or urgent revascularization at 30 days.
    b. Stenting plus abciximab reduces mortality, MI, or urgent revascularization at 6 months.

c. Stenting plus abciximab reduces mortality at 1 year.
d. All of the above.

ANSWER: d

In the EPISTENT trial (Lancet 1998;352:87–92), the combination of stent plus abciximab resulted in decreased mortality, MI, or urgent revascularization at 30 days and at 6 months. Mortality was reduced at 1-year follow-up.

32.   A 68-year-old man is admitted to the hospital with an acute anterior wall MI. You see him in the emergency room. His BP is 135/80 mm Hg, his HR is 85 bpm, and his physical examination is unremarkable except for an S4 gallop at the apex. LAD is 100% occluded, RCA contains an 80% mid stenosis and ejection fraction is 35%. He undergoes primary PTCA and is hemodynamically stable and pain free. Which one of the following statements is TRUE regarding his outcome?

a. The use of intra-aortic balloon pump after primary PTCA will reduce the infarct-related artery reocclusion.
b. His overall clinical outcome will be improved by adjunctive intra-aortic balloon pump insertion.
c. Myocardial recovery will be hastened by the use of intra-aortic balloon pump.
d. His outcome is not going to be influenced by the prophylactic use of the intra-aortic balloon pump.

ANSWER: d

A prospective, randomized trial of prophylactic intra-aortic balloon pump insertion in hemodynamically stable high-risk patients failed to show improvement in individual endpoints or the primary combined endpoint of death, reinfarction, infarct-related artery reocclusion, stroke, new-onset heart failure, and sustained hypotension (PAMI II) (*J Am Coll Cardiol* 1997;29(7):1459–1467).

33.   A 73-year-old woman is admitted to the hospital with a chest pain syndrome of approximately 15 hours duration. Her ECG reveals an evolving inferior MI. All of the following measures are proven to improve her outcome, **EXCEPT:**

a. Full anticoagulation with heparin
b. Aspirin
c. β-Blockers
d. Cardiac catheterization and possible angioplasty

ANSWER: a

Despite being a common practice, the use of heparin for acute MI in patients treated with aspirin but not receiving thrombolytics has not proven to be of benefit. Furthermore, the current recommendations from both the American College of Physicians and the ACC/AHA are rather ambiguous except for a strong recommendation for high-risk patients (large anterior MI, severe left ventricular dysfunction, atrial fibrillation, and history of systemic or pulmonary embolism). A recent retrospective analysis revealed that the addition of heparin did not add any survival advantages and that perhaps the risk-benefit ratio may be unfavorable due to bleeding complications (*J Am Coll Cardiol* 1998;31:957–963).

Revascularization in this late presenting patient is perhaps best treated with angioplasty if there is evidence of ongoing ischemia (*Ann Intern Med* 1997;126:561–582). The risk-benefit ratio for thrombolytics increases with time, and beyond 12 hours it is probably not helpful.

34.   Which location is less predisposed to restenosis after angioplasty of SVG lesion?

     a. Mid vein graft
     b. Distal anastomotic site
     c. Proximal anastomotic site

ANSWER: b

The rate of restenosis after plain angioplasty of vein grafts depends on the location of the lesion as well as the age of the graft (*J Interven Cardiol* 1997;10:195–205). The proximal anastomotic site and mid graft lesions have the highest rate of restenosis after PTCA (60% to 70%). The distal anastomotic lesions have the best outcome in terms of restenosis rate (45%) and 5-year survival (92%).

Other revascularization techniques fail to result in lower rates of restenosis, but stenting offers higher success rate. The results of stenting do not depend on the age of the graft. The restenosis rate after stenting de novo graft lesions is about 20%, with an event-free survival at 1 year of 70% to 75% (*J Am Coll Cardiol* 1995;26: 704–712; *Am J Cardiol* 1994;74:1187–1191). However, the only randomized trial of stents versus PTCA in vein grafts did not show a "significant" reduction in restenosis. A larger sample size would likely have shown a significant difference.

The presence of reactive cells demonstrated by histologic studies of stents in venous graft lesions suggested that, unlike restenosis in native vessels, the restenotic process in vein graft conduits extends beyond 6 months.

35.   Of the following statements regarding SVGs, all are TRUE, **EXCEPT:**

   a. The native vessels should be treated whenever possible.
   b. Due to its length and flexibility, the Gianturco-Roubin stent is the stent of choice in treating SVGs.
   b. Multiple stent implantation is not predictive of increased risk of restenosis.
   d. TEC is associated with >10% risk of distal embolization and >60% restenosis rate.

ANSWER: b

Because of high restenosis rates and steady progression of disease in SVGs, whenever possible the native vessels should be treated for better long-term results.

There is no stent of choice for SVG lesions. Each stent design offers a particular advantage. Theoretically, stents with smaller gaps are likely to achieve better results in friable grafts, reducing the distal embolization. The radial force exerted by the stent may also be an important feature of the device for the treatment of fibrotic graft lesions. Palmaz-Schatz, Gianturco-Roubin, Wallstent, and Wiktor stents have been used successfully to treat graft lesions. While the Palmaz biliary stent offers increased resistance to radial compressive force, the Wiktor stent and newer stents offer flexibility and the Wallstent has the ability to entrap friable graft material within its mesh. Presently, there are little comparative data among different types of stents. The only comparative trial in vein grafts found similar results between the Wallstent and the Palmaz-Schatz stent.

The major predictors of restenosis of SVG lesions treated with stents are restenotic lesions, small graft diameter, diabetes mellitus, and significant residual stenosis. The number of implantable stents did not correlate with restenosis (*J Am Coll Cardiol* 1995;26:704–712), although studies with angiographic follow-up are limited.

TEC is associated with a 12% rate of distal embolization and a 69% restenosis rate (*Circulation* 1994;89:302–312). The device is helpful in debulking heavily thrombosed or totally occluded vessels.

36.   Which is the strongest predictor of stent thrombosis when stenting is used to treat acute MI?

    a. The thrombus burden at the lesion site
    b. Stent underexpansion
    c. Low plaque mass
    d. Use of oversized balloons

ANSWER: b

Stenting has been avoided in the setting of acute MI because of the concern of stent thrombosis which, in major randomized trials, occurred in 3% to 5% of patients despite intense anticoagulation (*J Am Coll Cardiol* 1997;10:226).

Use of IVUS has revealed that stent underexpansion because of deployment at low pressure and/or undersized balloons represents an important correlative of in-stent thrombosis. Using high-pressure poststent dilatation and postprocedure antiplatelet therapy, the risk of stent thrombosis is less than 1% to 2% (ISAR study) (*J Am Coll Cardiol* 1997;29:28–34).

37.   Of the following statements regarding PTCA for treatment of acute MI, all are TRUE, **EXCEPT:**

    a. The incidence of events (death, nonfatal reinfarction, and nonfatal disabling CVA) at 30 days is significantly lower in a PTCA-treated group compared to a thrombolytic group.
    b. The rate of major events (nonfatal reinfarction, death, and target vessel revascularization) is lower in PTCA patients treated with abciximab compared to placebo.
    c. There is no difference in outcome between patients in the PTCA group treated with heparin versus those treated with hirudin.
    d. The ratio of TIMI 3 flow is higher after primary PTCA than after tPA.

ANSWER: b

In the GUSTO-IIb trial, 1138 patients were randomized to primary angioplasty or to accelerated tPA. One thousand twelve patients were randomly assigned to heparin or hirudin treatment. The primary study endpoint was a composite of death, nonfatal reinfarction, and nonfatal disabling stroke at 30 days. The primary endpoint was observed in 10.6% of patients in the angioplasty group assigned to heparin and in 8.2% of those assigned to hirudin ($P=0.37$) (*N Engl J Med* 1997;336:1621–1628). The incidence of the primary endpoint in the angioplasty and tPA group was 9.6% and 13.7%, respectively ($P=0.033$). Likewise, the PAMI study (*N Engl J Med* 1993;328:673–679) and meta-analysis of 10 randomized trials (*JAMA* 1997;279:2093–2098) showed benefits in these endpoints.

Although in a retrospective analysis abciximab was thought to be particularly helpful in MI patients, the only large prospective randomized trial (RAPPORT) in primary PTCA patients found no benefit in the primary endpoint of death, MI, or target vessel revascularization. The CADILLAC trial will complete enrollment in the autumn of 1999, and will determine which of the four strategies (PTCA versus stenting, abciximab versus no abciximab) is most effective in AMI patients.

Primary angioplasty studies have consistently shown higher rates of TIMI 3 flow compared to thrombolytic-treated patients (*N Engl J Med* 1996;335:1313–1317).

38.   Which of the following statements regarding the presence of coronary artery thrombus are TRUE?

    a. Angiography underestimates the presence of intravascular thrombus.
    b. There is a clear relationship between angiographic presence of thrombus and angioplasty outcome.
    c. Abciximab reduces the rate of adverse outcomes only in the cases when coronary thrombus is evident by angiography.
    d. The presence of thrombus is a contraindication to stenting because of increased risk of subacute thrombosis.

ANSWER: a

I.C. thrombus is seen frequently on angiographies of patients with acute coronary syndromes, and was seen as a contributor to an adverse outcome in an era when interventionalists did not use ticlopidine, stents, abciximab, and ACT-guided administration of heparin. The compared angioscopic and angiographic studies showed that angiography underestimates the presence of thrombus (*Cathet Cardiovasc Diagn* 1994;33:323–329).

The presence of angiographic thrombi was not conclusively associated with adverse outcome (*Circulation* 1996;93:253–258); revascularization rate was the same at 6 months (17.2% versus 17%) (*Circulation* 1996;93:889–897). The rate of periangioplasty complications (death, MI, revascularization) at 30 days and 6 months was not enhanced by the presence of thrombus. Abciximab treatment reduces the rate of complications regardless of the presence of I.C. thrombus (*J Am Coll Cardiol* 1998; 31:31–36).

Primary stenting in acute MI was considered a contraindication because of the potential risk of acute thrombosis. The safety of stenting in acute MI is evaluated in the PAMI-stent trial (the pilot study results were published in *J Am Coll Cardiol* 1998;31:23–30). The rate of subacute thrombosis was 1.3%. Based on these data, use of stents in infarct-related artery seems to be safe and is probably indicated when dissection is present after balloon dilatation or when there is greater than 30% residual stenosis.

Presently, there are not enough data regarding routine stenting in all cases of acute MI.

39.   An 80-year-old woman presents with a 2-hour history of intense chest pain, ST segment elevation in II, III, aVF, and ST segment depression in V_1 through V_2. Her past medical history is significant for chronic atrial fibrillation on warfarin therapy and a stroke 3 months ago. The physical examination shows a 50 kg elderly woman with a BP of 140/80 mm Hg and an HR of 80 bpm.

40.   A 68-year-old woman comes to the emergency room with a 3-hour history of chest pain, ST segment elevation in V_1 through V_5. Her BP is 80/60 mm Hg and her HR is 120 bpm.

41.   A 65-year-old man presents to the emergency room with a 3-hour history of chest pain (8/10); the ECG shows 3.0 mm ST depression in II, III, aVF, and V_5 through V_6; his BP is 130/70 and his HR is 78 bpm. He is started on appropriate

medical therapy but 30 minutes later his chest pain and ECG changes have not resolved.

42.   A 70-year-old man presents to the emergency room with a 14-hour history of stuttering chest pain and 1 mm ST segment elevation in leads II, III, and aVF.

43.   A 35-year-old man presents to the emergency room with a 5-hour history of chest pain and ST segment elevation in leads II, III and aVF. His BP is 120/60 mm Hg and his HR is 42 bpm, in sinus with a 2:1 AV block.

    a. Angiography and possible angioplasty emergently
    b. Thrombolytic therapy
    c. Either therapy
    d. None of the above

ANSWERS: 39-a, 40-a, 41-a, 42-a, 43-c

According to the ACC/AHA recommendations (*J Am Coll Cardiol* 1996;28:1328–1428), primary angioplasty as an alternative to thrombolytic therapy is a class IIa "in patients who have a risk-of-bleeding contraindication to thrombolytic therapy."

Absolute contraindications to thrombolysis include:

- history of hemorrhagic stroke at any time; older strokes or cerebral vascular events within 1 year
- known intracranial neoplasm
- active internal bleeding (does not include menses!)
- suspected aortic dissection

Relative contraindications are:

- severe uncontrolled hypertension on presentation (BP >180/110 mm Hg);
- history of prior CVA or known intracerebral pathology not covered above;
- current use of anticoagulants in therapeutic doses (INR 2.0);
- known bleeding diathesis;
- recent trauma (within 2 to 4 weeks), including head trauma or traumatic or prolonged (>10 minutes) cardiopulmonary resuscitation, or major surgery (<3 weeks);
- noncompressible vascular punctures;

- recent (within 2 to 4 weeks) internal bleeding;
- for streptokinase: prior exposure (especially within 5 days to 2 years) or prior allergic reaction;
- pregnancy;
- active peptic ulcer;
- history of chronic, severe hypertension.

Based on these recommendations, the cases in questions 39, 40, 41, and 42 are best treated with primary angioplasty.

The case in question 43 can be treated with either thrombolytics or primary angioplasty if it can be performed in a timely fashion by individuals skilled in the procedure (>75 PTCA/year), and supported by experienced personnel in high volume centers (>200 PTCA/year).

44.   A 55-year-old man is admitted with unstable angina for the last 48 hours that is uncontrollable by medical treatment. The angiogram reveals subtotally occluded proximal LAD and faint left-to-left collaterals to the distal LAD. Which strategy is superior in reducing CK-MB leak during revascularization?

    a. Balloon angioplasty alone
    b. Stenting in addition to abciximab
    c. Stenting alone
    d. Bypass surgery

ANSWER: b

Preliminary results of the largest coronary stent randomized trial (EPISTENT) demonstrated a superior 30-day and 6-month outcome (death, MI, and target vessel revascularization) for stenting plus abciximab when compared to balloon angioplasty plus abciximab and to stent alone. Reduction in death and MI was most prominent in patients presenting with unstable angina within the last 48 hours. The most frequent side effect was bleeding. This can be reduced by using weight-adjusted heparin protocol and early sheath removal.

The ongoing Controlled Abciximab and Device Investigation to Lower Late Angioplasty Complications (CADILLAC) study addresses this issue in acute MI patients. CABG results in an elevation in cardiac enzymes in more than 40% of patients.

45.   Primary stenting in the setting of acute MI is associated with improved outcome.

    a. True
    b. False
    c. Unknown

ANSWER: a

The prospective PAMI-Stent pilot trial found that primary stenting for acute MI is feasible in 77% of patients undergoing primary PTCA, with a 98% procedural success. Among stented patients, 93% were event-free (alive, without reinfarction or TVR) at 30 days and 83% were event-free at 6 months (*J Am Coll Cardiol* 1998;31:23–30).

The PAMI Heparin Coated Stent Pilot Trial (*J Am Coll Cardiol* 1997;29:389A) showed the same improvement in clinical outcome.

The first randomized trial of primary PTCA versus primary stenting was published in 1998 (*Circulation* 1998;97:2502–2505). The 6-month cardiac event-free rates were 95% after primary stenting and 80% after primary PTCA. The difference in the endpoint resulted from reduced rates of reinfarction (1% versus 7%) and TVR (4% versus 17%) in the stent group, with no difference in mortality. The randomized stent PAMI trial showed reduced rates of restenosis and target vessel revascularization, but no effect on reinfarction.

46.   A 38-year-old multiparous woman presents to the hospital with a 3-hour history of chest pressure. She is 16 weeks pregnant. Her ECG shows ST segment elevation in V_1 through V_5. Her BP is 130/80 and HR is 90 bpm. Of the following statements, all are TRUE, **EXCEPT:**

    a. Her prognosis is better because she is above age 35.
    b. Catheterization is contraindicated at this time because the organogenesis is not yet completed.
    c. Her mortality ranges between 37% and 50%.
    d. Use of low-dose aspirin is safe during pregnancy.
    e. Pregnancy is a relative contraindication to thrombolytic therapy.

ANSWER: b

Acute MI typically occurs antepartum in multiparous women and postpartum in primiparous women.

In the absence of a clear clinical picture and diagnostic ECG changes, one should keep in mind that CK-MB levels may be elevated (they are found in the placenta and uterus).

The prognosis is worsened by age under 35 years, advanced pregnancy, delivery within 2 weeks of the MI, and cesarean section (23% mortality compared to 14% mortality with vaginal delivery).

The treatment with nitrates and β-blockers should be done cautiously to avoid hypotension. Low-dose aspirin is safe.

Thrombolytics can be used in ultra-high-risk MI cases, although they are generally considered a contraindication during pregnancy, and limited experience is available.

Angiography should be done only if angioplasty or CABG are envisioned. Catheterization should be avoided during the first 14 weeks of pregnancy; later in pregnancy organogenesis is completed (*Cathet Cardiovasc Diagn* 1997;42:38–43). A lead drape should be placed over the patient's abdomen and pelvis.

47.   You are performing an angioplasty of the proximal LAD in a 62-year-old male who had presented with resting angina and deep T wave inversion on the antero-septal leads on the ECG. Your visual estimation of the vessel diameter distal to the lesion is 3.25 mm, and a 3.5×15 mm stent (Crown; Cordis) is deployed at the lesion after initial balloon inflation with a 3.0 balloon with an excellent angiographic result. Which one of the following statements is TRUE?

   a. IVUS is indicated to determine stent apposition and the need for further balloon inflations.
   b. No further action is needed.
   c. The patient should not be given abciximab.
   d. Postdilate with a 3.5 mm noncompliant balloon.

ANSWER: b

Despite the fact that IVUS led to the use of high-pressure dilatation after stent deployment, it is unproven whether routine use of IVUS will reduce the incidence of stent thrombosis (already very low, <1%) or improve restenosis; several studies currently await long-term data in this regard (AVID, CRUISE, OPTICUS, and

SIPS). Until a positive impact on outcome is proven, IVUS cannot be recommended in the present clinical situation due to the added cost and time commitment.

The Crown stent comes mounted on a high-pressure balloon and requires no further balloon dilatation unless undersizing is observed.

EPISTENT trial showed better 30-day and 6-month clinical outcome for stenting plus abciximab.

48.   Patients with refractory unstable angina who are on medical therapy benefit from administration of Gp IIb/IIIa receptor antagonists.

   a. True
   b. False

ANSWER: a

The c7E3 Fab AntiPlatelet Therapy in Unstable Refractory Angina (CAPTURE) study (*Lancet* 1997;349:1429–1435) showed that this category of patients benefitted from administration of abciximab; the drug was started 18 to 24 hours before PTCA and continued until 1 hour after PTCA. There was a reduction at 30 days of combined endpoint of death, MI, and need for revascularization (11.3% versus 15.9%; *P*=0.012) at the expense of more frequent bleeding (3.8% versus 1.9%). The target ACT in this study was 300 seconds. The benefit noticed at 30 days was lost at 6 months.

Likewise, tirofiban was shown in the PRISM and PRISM PLUS trials, and integrilin in the PURSUIT trial, to reduce the combined endpoint.

49.   A 51-year-old male presenting with an anterior wall MI undergoes primary angioplasty with restoration in TIMI 3 flow in the vessel 2 hours after the beginning of symptoms. Left ventriculogram reveals anteroapical akinesis. ECHO performed 1 week later reveals normal left systolic function.

50.   A 55-year-old woman with class III angina undergoes a cardiac catheterization that reveals severe 3 vessel disease and ventricular systolic function with an ejection fraction of 25%. Three months after bypass surgery, she is angina-free and an ECHO reveals normal systolic function.

51.   A 53-year-old male presents 4 hours after the onset of an inferior wall MI. He reports several episodes of angina the day before that resolved each with sublingual nitroglycerin. Primary angioplasty is performed successfully and left ventriculogram reveals overall normal left ventricular function with mild inferior wall hypokinesis.

     a. Preconditioning
     b. Stunning
     c. Hibernation

ANSWERS: 49-b, 50-c, 51-a

Myocardial *stunning* is the mechanical dysfunction that persists after reperfusion despite the absence of irreversible damage and despite return of normal or near normal perfusion. The pathogenesis is multifactorial with two plausible hypotheses: the oxyradical hypothesis postulates generation of reactive oxygen species, and the calcium hypothesis postulates alterations in the cellular calcium homeostasis that eventually create a disturbance of the myofilament function (*Circulation* 1998;97:1848–1867).

During angioplasty, brief occlusions (<60 seconds) are associated with persistent abnormalities in ventricular compliance (*J Am Coll Cardiol* 1986;7:455–461) and longer inflations (5 to 7 minutes) require 24 to 36 hours for full recovery of regional wall motion; this was improved with calcium channel blockade (*Am J Cardiol* 1995;75:22E–30E).

Hibernating myocardium represents reduced ventricular function in the setting of chronic reduced coronary blood flow that improves after coronary revascularization. The time course of recovery is variable and probably depends on the duration, severity of ischemia, and degree of revascularization. The pathogenesis is controversial between a metabolic adaptation (downregulation of oxygen consumption) and repetitive stunning.

Preconditioning refers to the ability of the myocardium that has been exposed to ischemia to better tolerate a more prolonged episode of ischemia than myocardium not previously exposed. There are certain limits, as the protection is transient and dissipates after 1 to 2 hours of reperfusion. In addition, if the duration of the ischemia is very long (>90 minutes in some models), then the benefits are lost. The definition has also been extended to include protection against arrhythmias and postischemic left ventricular dysfunction (stunning) (*Am J Cardiol* 1995;75:17A–25A).

There is a second window of protection 24 hours after a preconditioning stimulus of brief repetitive episodes of ischemia; it may extend up to 3 days. The mechanism is under investigation. This has been proven in the clinical setting (*Circulation* 1995;91: 37–47).

52.   Of the following statements regarding the peripheral vascular complications of coronary interventions, all are TRUE, **EXCEPT:**

    a. Arteriovenous fistula may appear in 0.1% to 1.5% of cases.
    b. Retroperitoneal hemorrhage is usually due to a high femoral arterial puncture.
    c. Accurate puncture of profunda femoris artery would prevent most cases of pseudoaneurysm formation.
    d. Arteriovenous fistulae that do not close by 2 to 4 weeks should be surgically repaired.

ANSWER: c

The most common complications after coronary interventions are:

- *Retro-peritoneal hemorrhage,* which is usually due to high femoral arterial puncture. The treatment is conservative at first: I.V. fluids, blood transfusions, removal of the arterial sheath, cessation of anticoagulant, prolonged compression, and bedrest. The best way to avoid this complication is to avoid entry of the common femoral artery near or above the inguinal ligament.
- *Arteriovenous fistulae* are usually due to a low puncture (of the superficial or profunda, transecting a small venous branch). They may complicate 0.1% to 1.5% of coronary interventions. Clinically, there may be a continuous bruit or edema. If the arteriovenous fistula does not close in 2 to 4 weeks, surgical repair or ultrasound-guided compression is recommended.
- *Pseudoaneurysms* are due to anticoagulation and inadequate compression following the sheath removal. If it is greater than 3.0 cm, ultrasound-guided compression

or surgical repair is recommended. As a general approach to common femoral artery puncture, fluoroscopic localization of the skin nick to overlie the inferior border of the femoral head will avoid the low or high inadequate punctures.

- *Cholesterol embolization* is discussed in another part of this manual.
- *Thrombotic occlusion* is more frequent with radial or brachial approach.
- *Hematoma and free bleeding* are treated on an individual basis.

53.   All of the following items are manifestations of cholesterol embolization syndrome, **EXCEPT:**

    a. Livedo reticularis
    b. Absent distal pulses
    c. Reduced complement level
    d. Renal failure
    e. Amaurosis fugax
    f. Abdominal pain

ANSWER: b

Cholesterol embolization is due to distal showering of cholesterol crystals from ulcerated plaques in the aorta, iliac arteries, or femoral arteries. The cholesterol crystals obstruct small peripheral arteries, resulting in ischemia and necrosis.

Any instrumentation of the aorta may result in atheromatous embolization. The manifestations of this syndrome are:

- Cutaneous: livedo reticularis, gangrene ("blue toe syndrome"), cyanosis, ulceration.
- Renal failure due to renal emboli. It can be associated with hypertension and may be irreversible.
- Central nervous system manifestations: amaurosis fugax, diffuse encephalopathy.
- Mesenteric embolization: abdominal pain, gastrointestinal bleeding, pancreatitis.
- Laboratory abnormalities: reduced complement level, eosinophilia, elevated erythrocyte sedimentation rate.

The prognosis is poor, with high morbidity and mortality (*Angiology* 1987;38:769).

54. Of the following statements regarding ELCA, all are TRUE, **EXCEPT:**

   a. Randomized trials showed similar procedural success rates and acute complication rates for PTCA and ELCA.
   b. Laser technique can be used for total occlusions that cannot be crossed with regular guiding wire and/or balloon.
   c. Presently, ELCA is not used as a "stand alone" procedure, but as an adjunctive to PTCA or stenting.
   d. At long-term follow-up there is no difference in event-free survival rate between PTCA and ELCA.

ANSWER: a

Randomized trials showed similar procedural success rate for PTCA and ELCA. The AMRO study (*Circulation* 1995;92:I-477), the ERBAC study (*Circulation* 1997;96:91–98), and the LAVA trial (*J Am Coll Cardiol* 1997;30:1714–1721) showed an increase in acute complication rate with ELCA. In the LAVA trial, 11-month follow-up showed the same event-free survival rate.

Presently, ELCA should not be considered a stand-alone procedure, but rather an adjunctive to PTCA and stenting. The device is potentially useful for chronic total occlusions (including use of laser wire for total occlusions which cannot be crossed with regular wire), aorto-ostial lesions, long lesions, and in-stent restenosis lesions.

55. A 25-year-old woman presents with initially moderate exertional dyspnea of 6 months duration. It has worsened over the last few weeks. Her physical examination reveals a II/IV late peaking systolic ejection murmur at the base—P2 was delayed. Two-dimensional ECHO reveals a 70 mm Hg systolic mean gradient across the pulmonary valve when measured by continuous wave Doppler; the infundibulum was not involved. The BEST initial treatment option is:

   a. Surgical valvotomy.
   b. Percutaneous balloon valvuloplasty with the Inoue balloon catheter (Toray Medical Co., Ltd., Tokyo, Japan).
   c. Percutaneous balloon valvotomy if there is evidence of a dysplastic valve.
   d. If the infundibulum is affected, valve replacement is preferred.

ANSWER: b

Percutaneous valvuloplasty is the treatment of choice for congenital pulmonary stenosis in children. In adults and adolescents the procedure can be performed safely, and long-term results appear to be similar to those in young children. It also has been performed in infundibular stenosis and this is no longer regarded as a contraindication for pulmonary valvuloplasty. However, the presence of dysplastic valves requires a surgical approach.

The Inoue balloon is preferred because it is flexible and short, thus minimizing injury to the outflow tract and main pulmonary artery. Moreover, it is self-positioning and the adjustable inflation makes a stepwise dilation possible with a single balloon. Finally, it has a short inflation-deflation cycle that allows minimal hemodynamic compromise (*N Engl J Med* 1996;335:21–25).

56.   Of the following statements regarding adult patients with mitral stenosis (mitral valve area ≤1.5 cm²), all are TRUE, **EXCEPT:**

   a. Percutaneous trans-septal mitral valvotomy is currently the initial treatment of choice for symptomatic patients.
   b. Open surgical commissurotomy is to be reserved for patients with unfavorable echocardiographic features.
   c. Restenosis after balloon valvotomy is estimated to be ~7E 40% to 50%.
   d. The rate of residual atrial septal defect after balloon valvotomy is 10%.

ANSWER: c

In recent studies with a follow-up of 3 years, the restenosis rate for balloon valvotomy is approximately 12%. This is similar to that of closed surgical commissurotomy (*N Engl J Med* 1994;331: 961–967).

Echocardiographic features that favor surgery include severe calcification and thickening of the valvular and subvalvular apparatus, and lack of mobility.

In addition, NYHA class IV, elevated left ventricular end-diastolic pressure and associated significant mitral regurgitation also favor surgery (*N Engl J Med* 1992;327:1329–1335).

57. Aortic balloon valvuloplasty is recommended in all of the following clinical scenarios, **EXCEPT:**

  a. Symptomatic aortic stenosis in patients whose life expectancy is <1 to 2 years due to severe comorbid illness.
  b. Advanced age.
  c. As a "bridge" to surgery in patients whose hemodynamic instability makes them unacceptable for surgery in the present condition.
  d. Patients with moderate to severe left ventricular systolic dysfunction and a low aortic gradient and cardiac output where valvuloplasty MAY be used to determine whether the patient may benefit from valve replacement.

ANSWER: b

Age alone should NOT be used as a deferring reason for elective aortic valve replacement. The long-term results of aortic balloon valvuloplasty have been poor (mortality 45% at 1 year) (*Circulation* 1994;89:642); thus aortic balloon valvuloplasty should only be used in those above mentioned situations and after exhaustive discussion among all involved.

58. Of the following statements regarding IMA conduit, all are TRUE, **EXCEPT:**

  a. Long-term patency of IMA grafts to vessels with <50% stenosis is lower than to vessels with more significant lesions.
  b. Perioperative anterior wall ischemia after LIMA placement is most frequently related to acute graft thrombosis secondary to artery manipulation.
  c. Long-term patency rates for LIMA to LAD are approximately 95%.
  d. The patency rate is improved if the vessel distal to the anastomotic site is free of occlusions worse than 25% of the lumen.

ANSWER: b

Perioperative ischemia of the anterior wall is rare after LIMA to LAD and is probably due to diffuse spasm of the graft; it is treated with nitrates (nitroglycerin, nitroprusside) and verapamil (*J Thorac Cardiovasc Surg* 1994;107:1440).

Patency rates of IMA to coronary arteries with stenosis less than 50% are lower than in those with stenosis greater than 50% (the pressure gradient across a stenosis <50% is minimal).

Long-term patency rates for IMA to LAD, LCX, and RCA are 95%, 88%, and 76%, respectively.

The patency is improved if the distal run-off is free of stenoses (≤25% of vessel lumen) and the vessel diameter is ≥1.5 cm.

59.   A 49-year-old man underwent heart transplantation 3 years ago. He did well until recently, when he started to experience exertional dyspnea. A nuclear exercise stress test was positive for reversible anterior wall ischemia. Of the following statements, all are TRUE, **EXCEPT:**

   a. Coronary disease develops by 5 years in almost half of patients.
   b. The best way to follow up these patients would be to do annual imaging stress tests.
   c. PTCA is not recommended in transplant patients.
   d. A history of graft rejection and cytomegalovirus (CMV) infection increases the risk of developing coronary disease.

ANSWER: c

New-onset coronary disease can complicate heart transplantation. By 5 years, 40% of patients have significant coronary stenoses. Because the transplanted heart is denervated, these patients will not have angina when they are ischemic; the best form of follow-up would be an annual imaging stress test.

If the stress test suggests significant coronary occlusion, angiography should be performed, followed by PTCA if necessary.

The coronary stenoses in this category of patients are due probably to an immunologic response; a history of repeated rejection episodes or CMV infection increases the risk of developing coronary disease, which, as opposed to native vessels, is more diffuse, distally located, and is associated with less lipid accumulation.

60.   Of the following statements concerning treatment of calcific lesions, all are TRUE, **EXCEPT:**

   a. Rotablator atherectomy of calcific and noncalcific lesions result in equivalent procedural success rates.

  b. The procedural success for rotational atherectomy is superior to that for PTCA of calcific lesions.
  c. A stepped burr approach is not necessary in this particular type of lesion because of the very low risk of perforation.
  d. Undersizing the first burr is recommended in heavily calcified lesions.

ANSWER: c

Rotational atherectomy is the procedure of choice for treatment of calcific lesions. The success rate is similar to that of noncalcific lesions and higher when compared to PTCA for calcific stenoses (ERBAC study final results [abstract] *J Am Coll Cardiol* 1994; 23[2]:57A).

A stepped burr-size approach is recommended. For heavily calcified lesions a small burr can be used initially in order to decrease the distal plaque embolization.

61.   Which of the following statements regarding PTCA versus medical therapy in a patient with stable angina and one vessel disease is TRUE?

  a. PTCA will offer better survival at 6 months.
  b. PTCA will reduce the risk of MI.
  c. PTCA will improve this patient's exercise performance at 6 months.
  d. PTCA will not offer any advantage over medical therapy.

ANSWER: c

The Angioplasty Compared with Medication Evaluation (ACME) study (*N Engl J Med* 1992;326:10–16) compared PTCA with medical therapy for single vessel disease and stable angina. At 6 months, PTCA offered better symptom control and improved exercise capacity (2.1 minutes compared to the baseline) over medical therapy (0.5 minutes; *P*<0.001). The results were maintained at 3-year follow-up.

The medically treated patients needed more revascularization procedures.

There were no differences in the rates of death or MI.

62.   Your noninterventional partner sends to you a 45-year-old woman with mitral stenosis and an ECHO score of 6. She has been in atrial fibrillation for 2 months. She has had a prior surgical commissurotomy. What should you do next?

a. Schedule her for catheterization and an ad hoc percutaneous mitral valvuloplasty.
b. Call your partner and ask if the ECHO showed right atrial thrombi and/or mitral regurgitation.
c. Send her back for medical treatment.
d. Call the surgeon to evaluate her for mitral valve replacement.

ANSWER: b

The ECHO score is calculated taking into account leaflet mobility and thickening, subvalvular apparatus thickening, and calcification (a score of 1 to 4 is given for each characteristic). A good candidate should have a score less than 8, young age, and normal sinus rhythm; a poor candidate is a patient older than 70, in chronic atrial fibrillation, who has a score greater than 11. Two important pieces of information regarding the ECHO are: presence of mitral regurgitation (which will make the patient a good candidate for mitral valve replacement) and presence of right atrial thrombi. After the surface ECHO confirms that the patient is a candidate, transesophageal ECHO is recommended to rule out left atrial thrombus. If thrombus is present, systemic anticoagulation is initiated and the patient is reassessed with transesophageal ECHO in 2 months.

Immediate complications of the procedure include severe mitral regurgitation, tamponade, residual atrial septal defect, and embolization. The restenosis rate is 5% to 10%.

Patients with prior surgical commissurotomy have similar results to those without previous surgery.

The success rate in de novo versus prior commissurotomized stenotic valves is the same with balloon valvuloplasty.

63.   Of the following statements regarding rotablator atherectomy, all are TRUE, **EXCEPT:**

a. The procedural success rate with rotablator atherectomy is increased by the adjunctive use of balloon angioplasty.
b. Restenosis rate is lower with rotablator than with angioplasty because of better debulking.
c. Patients with left ventricular dysfunction undergoing rotablator atherectomy may benefit from intra-aortic balloon pump insertion.
d. The target vessel revascularization rate may be increased by using excessive debulking.

ANSWER: b

Restenosis rate of rotablation atherectomy (57%) tends to be higher than PTCA (47%; $P=0.14$) (ERBAC study) (*Circulation* 1997;96:91–98), and target vessel revascularization is also higher (42.4% versus 31.9%; $P=0.01$).

The best results with regard to restenosis were obtained for short calcific stenoses; long lesions and/or noncalcific lesions had higher risk of restenosis (*J Am Coll Cardiol* 1995;25:95A).

The nonrandomized multicenter investigation of the rotablation atherectomy involving 2953 patients and 3717 treated lesions, showed that the procedural success rate (defined as <50% residual stenosis in the absence of death, Q wave MI, or emergency CABG) with rotablation is 85% and increased to 95% by adjunctive use of PTCA.

The lowest rates of target vessel revascularization procedures were seen when the burr-to-artery ratio was approximately 79% to 80%; minimal or excessive debulking result in higher restenosis rate (*J Am Coll Cardiol* 1996;27:291A).

64.   A 68-year-old man has a history of documented CAD and stable angina pectoris. He is evaluated by his cardiologist for silent ischemia with ambulatory ECG monitoring. Of the following statements regarding this patient, all are TRUE, **EXCEPT:**

    a. If the ambulatory ECG monitoring shows episodes of nocturnal asymptomatic ischemia, this patient probably has 2- or 3-vessel disease.
    b. The presence of silent ischemia would put this patient at a higher risk for subsequent events.
    c. Ambulatory monitoring of myocardial ischemia is a screening test for significant CAD.
    d. Atenolol treatment is indicated in this patient.

ANSWER: c

There are two types of silent myocardial ischemic events: *type I* (in which patients do not experience angina at any time) and *type II* (occurring in patients who have angina but who also have episodes of silent ST depression on ambulatory ECG monitoring). Type II silent ischemia can occur in patients with stable or unstable angina; nocturnal episodes of silent myocardial ischemia are associated with increased incidence of 2- or 3-vessel disease.

The presence of silent myocardial ischemia is of prognostic significance; it is associated with higher risk of cardiac events in patients with history of CAD (*Am J Cardiol* 1992;69:579). Exercise-induced ST segment depression is associated with increased cardiac mortality compared with that in patients who do not experience such episodes (*J Am Coll Cardiol* 1989;14:556).

The exercise stress test is the most important screening test for significant CAD; it identifies the majority of patients who might have asymptomatic ischemia during daily activities.

The Atenolol in Silent Ischemia Trial (ASIST) (*Am J Cardiol* 1994;74:1095) showed that silent myocardial ischemia can be suppressed; there was a significant decrease in the rate of coronary events (death, nonfatal MI, worsening angina) at 1 year in the atenolol-treated group compared to the placebo group.

65.   In your opinion, revascularization for the patient described above will:

   a.   Reduce the rate of hospital admissions
   b.   Reduce the rate of death
   c.   Reduce the rate of death or nonfatal MI
   d.   All of the above

ANSWER: d

The Asymptomatic Myocardial Ischemia pilot study compared the outcome of 558 patients with silent myocardial ischemia randomized to 3 treatment strategies: angina-guided drug therapy (n=183), angina plus ischemia-guided drug therapy (n=183), or revascularization by angioplasty or bypass surgery (n=192). Two years after randomization, the total mortality was 6.6% in the angina-guided strategy, 4.4% in the ischemia-guided strategy, and 1.1% in the revascularization strategy ($P<0.02$). The rate of death or MI was 12.1% in the angina-guided strategy, 8.8% in the ischemia-guided strategy, and 4.7% in the revascularization strategy ($P<0.04$). The rate of death, MI, or recurrent hospitalization was 41.8% in the angina-guided strategy, 38.5% in the ischemia-guided strategy, and 23.1% in the revascularization strategy ($P<0.001$) (*Circulation* 1997;95:2037–2043).

66.   Which one of the following patients would NOT benefit from carotid revascularization?

   a.   A patient with amaurosis fugax and 70% to 80% carotid stenosis.
   b.   An asymptomatic patient with 70% to 80% carotid stenosis.
   c.   A patient with a recent transient ischemic attack and a 30% carotid stenosis.
   d.   An asymptomatic patient with an absolute peak velocity of 110 cm/s at end diastole at the site of a 60% to 70% stenosis by duplex ultrasound.

ANSWER: c

The North American Symptomatic Carotid Endarterectomy Trial (NASCENT) and the Asymptomatic Carotid Artery Stenosis (ACAS) study, showed a benefit from surgical treatment of asymptomatic patients with greater than 70% carotid artery stenosis and symptomatic patients with greater than 60% carotid stenosis.

When Doppler ultrasound is used to evaluate the degree of stenosis, the most sensitive indicator is the *absolute peak velocity at the end diastole* at the site of the stenosis. A severe stenosis will be strongly suggested by a peak velocity of greater than 100 cm/s. The patient presented in item **d** needs an angiography to definitively evaluate the stenosis.

67.   Of the following statements regarding the stent thrombosis, all are TRUE, **EXCEPT:**

   a.   The incidence of subacute thrombosis is 0.5% to 1.0%.
   b.   Acute stent thrombosis in the catheterization laboratory is associated with the highest rate of ischemic complications.
   c.   Subacute thrombosis rate peaks at 3 to 5 days.
   d.   The risk of stent thrombosis is lower in SVGs than in native vessels.

ANSWER: b

The incidence of acute stent thrombosis is rare in the catheterization laboratory but can usually be treated quickly without significant clinical complications. It is the result of uncovered dissections, incomplete stent deployment, stenting in arteries with a diameter ≤3.0 mm, or persistent filling defects inside the stent. Stent thrombosis is rare after 2 weeks.

The new antiplatelet therapy (*N Engl J Med* 1996;334:1084–1089) and adjunctive high-pressure balloon dilatation (*Circulation*

1995;91:1676–1688) have reduced the incidence of stent thrombosis to less than 1%.

The bigger diameter of the SVGs is probably responsible for the lower rate of stent thrombosis.

68.   Of the following statements regarding residual dissection after stent placement, all are TRUE, **EXCEPT:**

    a. All dissections should be covered with stents, as their presence increases the risk of subacute thrombosis.
    b. Dissections left uncovered at the end of the stent do not increase the risk of restenosis.
    c. I.C. spasm may mimic a dissection at the end of the stent.

ANSWER: a

It was noted that stent deployment may cause small tears at the margins of the stent. The Stent Treatment Region assessed by Ultrasound (STRUT) registry showed that the frequency of edge dissections is ~12%.

The need for additional stenting in order to cover a dissection at the end of the stent should be a decision taken on a case-by-case basis: IVUS use showed that small tears at the edges of a stent do not have any clinical significance (*Circulation* 1995;92:I-546). A large, mobile flap with blood speckling behind the tear or a long dissection in a large vessel should be treated with stent deployment; one should keep in mind, though, that additional stenting increases the risk of acute thrombosis and restenosis. Therefore, the additional stenting should be used on a case-by-case basis.

Coronary spasm, wire-induced pseudolesions, plaque shifting, and wall calcification may mimic dissection.

Dissections do not increase the risk of restenosis (*Circulation* 1995;92:I-546).

69.   Potential revascularization options for patients who are not amenable to percutaneous or surgical means because of poor distal run-off and lack of targets include:

    a. External counterpulsation
    b. Surgical transmyocardial laser revascularization (TMR)

c. Percutaneous TMR
d. Angiogenesis via delivery of growth factors
e. All of the above

ANSWER: e

With TMR it was thought that the creation of microchannels would serve as an "artificial Tebesian system," whereby blood would flow from the ventricular cavity directly into the myocardium. It has, however, been demonstrated that these channels do not remain patent. It is possible that they induce neovasculature. Improvements in angina class have been seen in patients with end-stage CAD (*J Thorac Cardiovasc Surg* 1997;113:645–654). Percutaneous approaches are being investigated, but not enough clinical data are yet available (*Circulation* 1997;96[suppl I]:I-218). According to the Food and Drug Administration, 72% of angina patients treated with TMR in trials had significant reduction in angina pain in the first year compared to 13% of patients treated with conventional medical treatment. TMR timing is essential; it should not be used in patients who have recently had an MI, or in those likely to have an MI in the next 6 weeks after surgery.

The administration of vascular endothelial growth factors such as the fibroblast growth factor-1 (FGF-1 acidic) appears promising (*Circulation* 1998;97:645–650).

External enhanced counterpulsation (EECP) has shown a reduction in angina events, in perfusion defects evaluated by nuclear studies, and in hospitalization rates. One possible explanation, although speculative, for the improvement in the perfusion is that EECP may open or enhance collateral channels when at least one patent conduit (native vessel or graft) is present. It requires several sessions (up to 35 one-hour visits) (ACC 47th Annual Scientific Session, March 1998).

70.   Of the following statements regarding TEC atherectomy, all are TRUE, **EXCEPT:**

a. This device was designed to extract thrombi and therefore its use in SVGs eliminates the risk of distal embolization.
b. A "dotter" effect contributes to some of the angiographic improvement after TEC atherectomy.
c. The presence of thrombus does not influence the success rate.
d. Calcified lesions are a contraindication to TEC atherectomy.
e. TEC atherectomy is superior to PTCA for reducing periprocedural CK-MB elevations.

ANSWER: a

TEC is used successfully to remove thrombus from venous graft conduits; there is a high risk of distal embolization and "no reflow" after the use of the device in highly thrombotic, old, friable grafts. In TEC Multicenter Registry data, the rates of distal embolization and no reflow were 11.9% and 8.8%, respectively.

In one study, histologic examination of the material extracted with TEC did not show tissue particles; it was speculated that mechanical dilatation rather than plaque removal contributes to the angiographic improvement after TEC (*J Interven Cardiol* 1993;5: 31–39). However, current techniques using prolonged suction and multiple vacuum bottles at the lesion extract multiple atherosclerotic particles.

The TEC Registry showed that the presence of thrombus does not decrease the rate of initial success when TEC atherectomy is used.

Certain lesions, including bifurcation, eccentric, severely angulated, calcified lesions as well as lesions in small vessels, are considered contraindicated to TEC atherectomy.

The randomized TOPIT trial, which was conducted in post-MI or unstable angina patients found that TEC atherectomy was associated with a reduction in new CK elevations compared to PTCA.

71.   Of the following statements regarding intracoronary thrombus, all are TRUE, **EXCEPT:**

   a. Rheolytic thrombectomy is a promising technique for thrombus removal.
   b. Urokinase is more effective than tPA and streptokinase for treating intracoronary thrombus.
   c. Stent thrombosis can be successfully treated with I.C. thrombolytics or Gp IIb/IIIa receptor antagonist alone.
   d. I.C. thrombolytics are useful in treating total chronic occlusions in native vessels or vein grafts.
   e. No reflow is not an indication for I.C. thrombolytics.

ANSWER: c

Stent thrombosis is an emergency that requires diagnostic cardiac catheterization followed by PTCA. Lytics or abciximab can be used if necessary as adjunctive to interventional procedure.

Rheolytic thrombectomy is promising but is still an investigational tool for treating I.C. thrombosis.

For selective intra-arterial thrombolysis there is a general consensus that urokinase is more effective than streptokinase and tPA; however, randomized comparisons are lacking and adjunctive thrombolytics may worsen the procedural outcome.

Although rarely used nowadays, I.C. administration of thrombolytics for chronic total occlusions is an accepted therapeutic method that results in angiographic improvement at the price of relatively low risk (MI, early and late reocclusion, bleeding). It consists of placing an infusion catheter proximal to the lesion.

Distal microembolization, characteristically manifested as "no re-flow," is treated successfully in most cases with I.C. calcium antagonists or adenosine.

72.   A patient who received a 3.0 mm stent 6 months ago comes back with angina and in-stent restenosis is demonstrated. You decide to debulk the lesion using rotablation atherectomy. What would be the maximum recommended burr size?

    a.   1.5 mm
    b.   1.75 mm
    c.   2.0 mm
    d.   2.25 mm

ANSWER: d

The technique used for rotablation atherectomy of diffuse in-stent restenosis is a step approach, starting with a small burr (especially in treating total occlusions when the intraluminal position of the distal wire is uncertain); the final burr should be 70% of the stent diameter (in this case, 2.25 mm burr). The stepped approach is not necessary if the lesion is focal. IVUS can be helpful in guiding burr size.

73.   The randomized trials of PTCA versus CABG have the following limitation(s):

    a.   Only a small number of patients who were suitable were randomized.
    b.   Long-term follow-up was limited to less than 6 years.
    c.   Many surgical complications were not considered in the follow-up.
    d.   Stents and minimally invasive surgery were not used.
    e.   All of the above.

ANSWER: e

The 6 large randomized trials (see below) that compared CABG with PTCA have a few limitations. A total of 4772 patients were enrolled; only 4% to 7% were suitable for randomization. The follow-up was limited to less than 6 years; a longer follow-up could have made a difference due to appearance of late disease in bypass grafts. Surgical complications (stroke, transfusion, pulmonary emboli, pain, non Q wave MI) were not considered as an endpoint. New percutaneous revascularization techniques and minimally invasive surgery were not available during the enrollment period of these studies.

03/1993: The Randomized Intervention Trial of Angina (RITA)

10/1993: The Argentine Randomized Trial of PTCA versus CABG in multivessel diseases (ERACI)

10/1994: The Emory Angioplasty versus Surgery Trial (EAST)

10/1994: The German Angioplasty Bypass Surgery Intervention Trial (GABI)

11/1995: The Coronary Angioplasty versus Bypass Revascularization Investigation (CABPRI)

07/1996: The Bypass Angioplasty Revascularization Investigation (BARI)

74.   The question of PTCA/stent implantation versus CABG for multivessel disease is not answered as of yet.

    a. True
    b. False

ANSWER: a

There are a few up and coming randomized trials that are trying to answer to this question:

 • The ARTS trial conducted by Serruys in Rotterdam.
 • The SOS trial is led by Ulrich Sigwart in the U.K.
 • The multicenter Stent Implantation versus Minimally Invasive Surgery (SIMIS) will compare both techniques.

The results of these trials will be available in the next few years.

75. Of the following statements regarding stenting, all are TRUE, **EXCEPT:**

    a. Elective stenting in de novo lesions results in less restenosis than stenting in restenotic lesions.
    b. The time frame of restenosis is absolutely the same for PTCA and stent.
    c. There is more intimal proliferation after stenting.
    d. Poststent residual stenosis of more than 10% is associated with increased risk of restenosis.

ANSWER: b

Restenosis after PTCA is rare in the first month, it plateaus at 3 to 6 months, and then it remains stable. In-stent minimal lumen diameter may actually improve between 6 months and 3 years (*J Am Coll Cardiol* 1995;25:375A).

76. Significant subclavian artery stenosis is defined as a systolic BP difference between the two arms of:

    a. 5 mm Hg
    b. 10 mm Hg
    c. 15 mm Hg
    d. 20 mm Hg

ANSWER: d

A systolic BP difference between the two arms of more than 20 mm Hg and reversal of flow in the ipsilateral vertebral artery are diagnostic for significant subclavian artery stenosis.

77. Which one of the following lesions of renal arteries is associated with higher rate of success and a lower restenosis rate?

    a. Fibromuscular dysplasia
    b. Atherosclerotic stenoses
    c. Ostial lesions
    d. Total occlusions

ANSWER: a

Fibromuscular dysplasia is associated with high rate of success and less restenosis. Athcrosclerotic lesions have higher rate of restenosis. Ostial lesions and total occlusions have low success rates.

Chapter 7

Statistics and Cost

QUESTIONS

1. Which one of the following options is the most cost effective?

   a. Use of low-osmolar, nonionic agents in all patients because the initial high cost will be offset by preventing complications secondary to contrast dye.
   b. Use ionic agents for all patients except those in renal failure.
   c. Use standard ionic agents for all elective cases and premedicate with steroids the patient allergic to contrast dye.
   d. Use low osmolar dye in patients with congestive heart failure or renal failure, or in those who have had a previous reaction to contrast agent.

2. Which one of the following statements comparing one-stage PTCA with staged procedure is **TRUE**?

   a. Ad hoc angioplasty consistently leads to an economic advantage over staged strategy.
   b. The risk of complications is significantly higher with ad hoc PTCA than with staged procedure in all groups of patients.
   c. There is a significant difference in the length of stay between one-stage PTCA and staged procedures.
   d. The cost advantage of ad hoc strategy is most likely to be realized when stenting is used.

3. Which definition of restenosis allows a more effective comparison between different types of coronary interventions?

   a. Continuous definition
   b. Dichotomous definition

4. Which of the following statements regarding abciximab is TRUE?

   a. Abciximab is beneficial only when used in high-risk

patients (MI within the previous week or an adverse lesion morphology on angiography).
b. The cost of a single dose of abciximab is approximately $2400.
c. The cost of a coronary revascularization procedure will be increased by use of abciximab and heparin, due to increased bleeding.
d. The net cost of abciximab at 6 months is approximately $1200 per patient.

5. Which one of the following statements regarding comparison between different types of stents is **FALSE**?

a. Palmaz-Schatz stent represents the gold standard against which all other stents are judged.
b. The goal of the equivalency trials between different stents was to show that new stents are comparable with Palmaz-Schatz stents for the primary endpoints of death, MI, and urgent revascularization.
c. The trials were designed to prove the superiority of one stent over another.
d. The second-generation stents offer secondary benefits.

Match the following:

6. Sensitivity

7. Specificity

8. Positive predictive value

9. Overall accuracy

10. Prevalence of a disease

a. The proportion of all patients with a disease from all patients tested.
b. Proportion of patients with true positive test results from the total patient population with positive test results.

c. Proportion of the subpopulation with disease that has a positive test.
d. The ratio of all true results (positive and negative) and the total number of tests performed.
e. Proportion of the subpopulation with no disease that has a negative test.

11.   Of the following statements regarding the cost-effectiveness (C/E) ratio, all are TRUE, **EXCEPT:**

a. The net cost of a procedure is part of C/E ratio calculation.
b. The economic value of a new medical treatment is assessed by using ranges of C/E ratios for other medical interventions.
c. Health benefits are best measured in terms of quality-adjusted life years (QALYs).
d. A C/E ratio of $50,000–60,000 per QALY is considered favorable in most medical systems.

12.   A patient has normal left ventricular function and one vessel disease (LAD). Which one of the following statements regarding this patient's treatment is **FALSE**?

a. If the patient has severe angina, QALY with initial percutaneous revascularization treatment is better than with initial medical therapy.
b. If the patient has mild angina, initial PTCA treatment will have an incremental C/E ratio of $20,000 to $40,000.
c. If the patient has severe angina, the C/E ratio is $6000 per QALY.

13.   Regarding the cost effectiveness of different revascularization procedures, all of the following statements are TRUE, **EXCEPT:**

a. Stenting for single vessel coronary artery disease has a cost effectiveness compared to that of treating mild diastolic hypertension.

b. Rotablation atherectomy, DCA, and ELCA are not cost effective compared to routine PTCA.
c. Primary angioplasty for patients with acute MI is probably cost effective if done in hospitals with 24-hour available cardiac catheterization laboratory and high procedural volume.
d. The 5-year cost effectiveness of PTCA for multivessel disease is lower when compared to CABG for multivessel disease.

14.   A pie chart format for data display is most useful when one wants to emphasize:

a. The results of two different types of medical treatment.
b. The percent with which each category contributes to the population as a whole.
c. Comparison of discrete variables.
d. That data are not intervally numeric, but ranked.

15.   In a comparison of PTCA and CABG for multivessel disease, there were important cost savings in the PTCA group; the difference was maintained at 5 years follow-up.

a. True
b. False

ANSWERS

1. Which one of the following options is the most cost effective?

    a. Use of low-osmolar, nonionic agents in all patients because the initial high cost will be offset by preventing complications secondary to contrast dye.
    b. Use ionic agents for all patients except those in renal failure.
    c. Use standard ionic agents for all elective cases and premedicate with steroids the patient allergic to contrast dye.
    d. Use low osmolar dye in patients with congestive heart failure or renal failure, or in those who have had a previous reaction to contrast agent.

ANSWER: d

The major drawback of the low-osmolar ionic and nonionic contrast agents is their significant increase in cost relative to standard ionic agents. The exclusive use of low osmolar contrast dye is associated with high cost and lack of clear benefit. A cost-effective policy would be to use low osmolar dye for most elective cases and low-osmolar, low-ionic dye for selected cases (patients with CHF, renal failure, or history of contrast dye allergy).

In patients with normal renal function, there is no advantage of using low-osmolar contrast dye over high osmolar contrast agents in an effort to prevent nephrotoxicity (*N Engl J Med* 1989; 320:149).

The following indications for use of low-osmolar contrast agents are currently accepted: CHF, renal insufficiency, hypotension, severe bradycardia, history of contrast allergy, severe valvular disease, IMA injection. The issue of nonionic agent-related thrombogenicity has risen, especially in patients with unstable coronary syndromes (unstable angina, acute MI) and hemodynamic compromise. A solution would be the use of a low-osmolality ionic agent (ioxaglate), which retains the anticoagulant properties of nonionic media. The disadvantage resides in the higher cost of such agents.

The existence of a large group of patients who derive no benefit from the use of low osmolar contrast agents emphasizes the need for selective rather than universal use of the more expensive agents. The high-risk patients will derive a commensurate safety benefit from the low osmolar agents, rendering their use justifiable.

2.   Which one of the following statements comparing one-stage PTCA with staged procedure is **TRUE**?

    a. Ad hoc angioplasty consistently leads to an economic advantage over staged strategy.
    b. The risk of complications is significantly higher with ad hoc PTCA than with staged procedure in all groups of patients.
    c. There is a significant difference in the length of stay between one-stage PTCA and staged procedures.
    d. The cost advantage of ad hoc strategy is most likely to be realized when stenting is used.

ANSWER: d

One-stage PTCA has become increasingly frequent in the last few years due to a number of factors including safer procedures in the setting of stent availability and, lately, abciximab use, as well as excellent digital images, which reduce the risk of erroneous reading.

Routine combined strategy for angiography and angioplasty is generally feasible, safe, and easier for the patient (*Am J Cardiol* 1995;75[1]:30–33; *J Am Coll Cardiol* 1998;31:321–325).

A cost advantage of ad hoc PTCA cannot be consistently demonstrated. Although some studies suggest that early PTCA may result in earlier patient discharge (*Am J Cardiol* 1995;75[1]:30–33), a recent study showed no difference in cost between the two strategies, with only one exception: for patients who received stents, in all cases an ad hoc strategy had significantly lower overall cost as compared with staged strategy (*J Am Coll Cardiol* 1998; 31:321–325).

There were trends toward lower costs with a one-stage PTCA in patients with stable angina, and toward lower costs with staged procedure for patients with unstable angina or for post-MI patients. Any modest trend toward complications is magnified by increase in cost. Hence, the cost advantage of an ad hoc strategy is most likely to be realized in settings associated with enhanced safety (stable coronary syndromes, coronary lesions suitable for stenting, use of Gp IIb/IIIa receptor inhibitors).

3.   Which definition of restenosis allows a more effective comparison between different types of coronary interventions?

    a. Continuous definition
    b. Dichotomous definition

ANSWER: a

The most common definition of restenosis is diameter stenosis greater than 50% at follow-up (*Am J Cardiol* 1987;60:39B–43B), based on animal measurements of coronary flow reserve. Hence, this definition of restenosis is seen as a dichotomous event: either present or absent. However, this definition is limited by the need to calculate percent stenosis using a "normal" reference segment when the vessel may be diffusely diseased. Moreover, little physiological difference is present between 49% (no restenosis and 51% (restenotic) lesions.

On the other hand, the continuous outcomes definition of restenosis assumes that the event occurs more or less in all treated lesions. The change in MLD follows a Gaussian distribution (*J Am Coll Cardiol* 1992;19:939–945). For the purpose of comparison between different coronary interventions, the use of change in MLD, or continuous measurement of MLD is more accurate.

4.   Which of the following statements regarding abciximab is TRUE?

    a. Abciximab is beneficial only when used in high-risk patients (MI within the previous week or an adverse lesion morphology on angiography).
    b. The cost of a single dose of abciximab is approximately $2400.
    c. The cost of a coronary revascularization procedure will be increased by use of abciximab and heparin, due to increased bleeding.
    d. The net cost of abciximab at 6 months is approximately $1200 per patient.

ANSWER: c

Subgroup analysis of the EPILOG trial (*N Engl J Med* 1997; 336:1689–1696) revealed that abciximab was beneficial in both high- and low-risk patients. There were no differences in the abciximab effect according to age, gender, or weight. The high-risk patients benefitted the most.

Treatment with abciximab has clinical effects, but the drug is expensive and may not be indicated in all patients. A formal economic analysis of EPIC trial (*Circulation* 1996;94:629–635) showed that the mean cost of a single abciximab dose was $1407. The cost increased even further due to bleeding complications. However, the subsequent decrease in hospitalizations, repeat revascularizations, and ischemic events resulted in a net 6-month cost of abciximab of $293 per patient. However, subsequent trials have not shown a decrease in need for repeat revascularization, and stenting has eliminated the advantage of reduced ischemia. Thus, with current use of abciximab, the net 6-month cost is likely to be much greater.

5.   Which one of the following statements regarding comparison between different types of stents is **FALSE**?

    a. Palmaz-Schatz stent represents the gold standard against which all other stents are judged.
    b. The goal of the equivalency trials between different stents was to show that new stents are comparable with Palmaz-Schatz stents for the primary endpoints of death, MI, and urgent revascularization.
    c. The trials were designed to prove the superiority of one stent over another.
    d. The second-generation stents offer secondary benefits.

ANSWER: c

The Palmaz-Schatz stent was unequivocally proven to reduce restenosis and the need for reintervention in the STRESS (*N Engl J Med* 1994;331:496–501) and BENESTENT (*N Engl J Med* 1994;331:489–495) randomized controlled trials versus PTCA. It therefore represents the gold standard against which the other stents are evaluated.

The goals of the equivalency trials were:

- to prove the second-generation stents' comparability with the gold standard tubular slotted stent for the primary endpoints of death, MI, and emergent revascularization;
- to prove that the secondary benefits they have (lower profile, greater flexibility, longer length, stronger balloons, or lower cost) are not outweighed by reduction in primary benefits.

These trials were not designed to prove the superiority of one stent over another. Three of these equivalency trials are the ASC Multi-link Clinical Equivalence Trial (ASCENT), Study of Microstent's Ability to Limit Restenosis Trial (SMART), and NIRVANA trial, evaluating NIR stent.

6.   Sensitivity

7.   Specificity

8.   Positive predictive value

9.   Overall accuracy

10.   Prevalence of a disease

    a.   The proportion of all patients with a disease from all patients tested.
    b.   Proportion of patients with true positive test results from the total patient population with positive test results.
    c.   Proportion of the subpopulation with disease that has a positive test.
    d.   The ratio of all true results (positive and negative) and the total number of tests performed.
    e.   Proportion of the subpopulation with no disease that has a negative test.

ANSWERS: 6-c, 7-e, 8-b, 9-d, 10-a

11.   Of the following statements regarding the cost-effectiveness (C/E) ratio, all are TRUE, **EXCEPT:**

    a.   The net cost of a procedure is part of C/E ratio calculation.
    b.   The economic value of a new medical treatment is assessed by using ranges of C/E ratios for other medical interventions.
    c.   Health benefits are best measured in terms of quality-adjusted life years (QALYs).
    d.   A C/E ratio of $50,000–60,000 per QALY is considered favorable in most medical systems.

ANSWER: d

The ratio between net cost and health benefits (measured in terms of QALYs) represents the C/E ratio (*Am J Cardiol* 1997;80[4A]: 39B–43B).

The cost effectiveness is assessed by comparison with the C/E ratios of other medical treatments:

- A C/E ratio less than $20,000 per QALY (for example, the treatment of hypertension or dislipidemias in patients with established coronary artery disease) is highly cost-effective.
- A C/E ratio of $20,000 to $40,000 per QALY is acceptable.
- A C/E ratio of greater than $60,000 has low cost effectiveness.

12.   A patient has normal left ventricular function and one vessel disease (LAD). Which one of the following statements regarding this patient's treatment is **FALSE**?

   a. If the patient has severe angina, QALY with initial percutaneous revascularization treatment is better than with initial medical therapy.
   b. If the patient has mild angina, initial PTCA treatment will have an incremental C/E ratio of $20,000 to $40,000.
   c. If the patient has severe angina, the C/E ratio is $6000 per QALY.

ANSWER: b

Initial PTCA treatment is cost effective for patients with normal left ventricular function, one vessel disease, and severe angina (reflected by a C/E ratio of $6000 and increase in QALY).

If the anginal symptoms are mild, the C/E ratio is high ($80,000 to $100,000) per QALY and, therefore, the medical treatment should be used first (*Heart* 1997;78[suppl 2]:7–10).

13.   Regarding the cost effectiveness of different revascularization procedures, all of the following statements are TRUE, **EXCEPT:**

   a. Stenting for single vessel coronary artery disease has a cost effectiveness compared to that of treating mild diastolic hypertension.
   b. Rotablation atherectomy, DCA, and ELCA are not cost effective compared to routine PTCA.
   c. Primary angioplasty for patients with acute MI is probably cost effective if done in hospitals with 24-hour available cardiac catheterization laboratory and high procedural volume.
   d. The 5-year cost effectiveness of PTCA for multivessel disease is lower when compared to CABG for multivessel disease.

ANSWER: d

Elective Palmaz-Schatz stenting for single vessel coronary disease has an incremental cost effectiveness of $30,000 to $40,000 per QALY, which is acceptable (*Am J Cardiol* 1997;80[10A]:3K–9K) and comparable with the treatment for mild diastolic hypertension.

The CAVEAT study (*N Engl J Med* 1993;329:221–227) and the ER-BAC study (*Circulation* 1997;96:91–98) did not show any improvement in clinical outcome when new devices were used (DCA, ELCA, rotablation atherectomy versus routine PTCA).

The cost effectiveness of primary angioplasty versus thrombolytic therapy for acute MI depends on the setting in which the procedure is performed (*J Am Coll Cardiol* 1996;28:882–889). Primary PTCA is likely to be cost effective in hospitals with a fully supported cardiac catheterization laboratory, performing more than 200 procedures per year (*J Am Coll Cardiol* 1997;30:1741–1750).

The analysis of the EAST (*Circulation* 1995;92:2831–2840) and BARI (*N Engl J Med* 1996;335:217–225) trials showed that, although the initial cost of PTCA is less than the cost of CABG, due to repeat hospitalizations and further need for revascularization, at 5 years the initial cost difference in the favor of PTCA is lost.

14.   A pie chart format for data display is most useful when one wants to emphasize:

    a.   The results of two different types of medical treatment.
    b.   The percent with which each category contributes to the population as a whole.
    c.   Comparison of discrete variables.
    d.   That data are not intervally numeric, but ranked.

ANSWER: b

The pie chart format is the best way to show the percent that each category contributes to the population as a whole.

15.   In a comparison of PTCA and CABG for multivessel disease, there were important cost savings in the PTCA group; the difference was maintained at 5 years follow-up.

    a. True
    b. False

ANSWER: a

There was a 35% cost savings in the PTCA group during hospitalization; at 5 years, the difference was only 5% between PTCA and CABG, but was still significant.

Chapter 8

Clinical Cases

QUESTIONS

Clinical Case 1. Ostial Stenosis

A 65-year-old man presents with unstable angina. LAO angiogram (Fig. CC1–1) of RCA shows ostial disease as well as a midvessel high-grade lesion. There is TIMI 3 flow in the vessel. What would be your strategy?

Discussion: Ostial RCA lesions are difficult to treat and debulking therapy has been advocated. However, in the setting of unstable angina, rotational atherectomy is relatively contraindicated because of the potential presence of thrombus. Placement of a stent after dilating an ostial lesion is definitely recommended, due to the high restenosis rate. IVUS might play a role in defining the amount of calcium present and the appropriate stent expansion.

The working view is of paramount importance in stenting ostial lesions. The stent should be positioned slightly outside the ostium, but not more than 1 mm; a stent mounted on a high-pressure balloon is preferable because subsequent coronary engagement with the guider, and possible trauma, can be avoided. Once the stent is deployed, care must be taken not to damage the stent with the guider. An angiogram should be performed in a subselective manner. To avoid the damage and to determine adequate ostial scaffolding by the stent.

This particular case was treated using a Sport wire and a 3.0/15 mm Quantum Ranger balloon inflated at both lesions, followed by

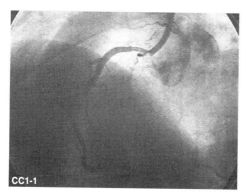

CC1-1

stenting with a 3.0/15 mm Multi-Link stent for the mid vessel and a 3.5/15 mm Multi-Link for the ostial lesion; both stents used were mounted on high-pressure balloons.

Clinical Case 2. Pseudolesion

LAO view of the RCA is shown (Fig. CC2–1) from a 60-year-old woman with post-MI angina. A high-torque intermediate wire was used, the lesion was crossed without difficulty, and a 2.5 Ranger balloon was inflated to nominal pressure at the lesion site. The wire was changed to an extrasupport wire. A 3.0/12 GFX stent (Arterial Vascular Engineering) was deployed at the lesion site; high-pressure balloon inflation was subsequently performed. The follow-up angiogram (Fig. CC2–2) is shown. What would you do next?

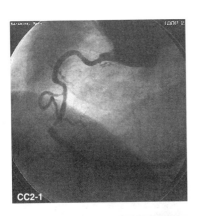

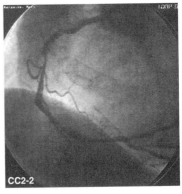

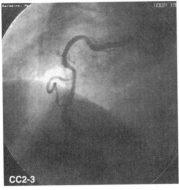

Discussion: The very tortuous coronary artery has straightened out with the stiffer wire and consequently, pseudolesions ("wrinkles") have developed; once the wire was pulled out, repeat angiogram (Fig. CC2–3) reveals disappearance of the pseudolesions. No further intervention was performed. If one is not entirely sure that the appearance is due to wrinkles, the wire may be partially retracted and only the radiopaque flexible end left at the site of the lesion, so that part of the wire is still across the lesion.

Clinical Case 3. Total Occlusion

A 52-year-old woman presents with a 2- to 3-month history of chest pain. A thallium stress test demonstrates reversible anterior wall ischemia at low work load. Coronary angiography reveals a total occlusion of the proximal LAD (Fig. CC3–1) and right-to-left collaterals. The other vessels are free of significant disease and the left ventricular function was normal. How would you approach this lesion?

Discussion: The following issues are essential in approaching this lesion.

    a. The lesion has favorable characteristics for a high success rate.

    b. The most important step in treating this lesion is atraumatic penetration of the lesion.

    c. Stenting this lesion is recommended.

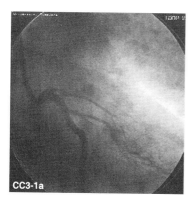 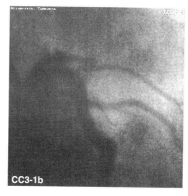

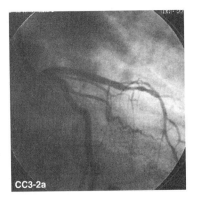
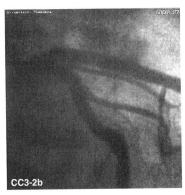

This patient is a very good candidate for percutaneous revascularization; she has a few of the angiographic characteristics of revascularization success:

- clinical duration of the symptoms less than 3 months;
- tapered stump;
- collaterals from the RCA;
- absence of "bridging collaterals";
- absence of wall calcification.

The key step in treating total occlusions is to place the wire in the distal vessel without inducing intimal trauma (dissection). The current approach is to start with softer wires (floppy) and advance gradually to stiffer wires (intermediate and standard). If these wires fail to cross the stenosis, a Magnum wire can be used. For total chronic occlusions, laser wire recanalization would be an alternative. If the lesion cannot be penetrated with any wire, maximal medical treatment should be tried before attempting more aggressive ways of revascularization.

Stenting is not mandatory if an acceptable result is obtained (residual stenosis ≤30%, without dissection). Given the high restenosis rate associated with total occlusions, primary stenting should be considered.

In this specific case, a high-torque floppy wire failed to cross the stenosis; a Choice extra-support wire (Boston Scientific/SciMed Inc., Watertown, MA) successfully penetrated the occlusion. A 3.5/15 mm Quantum Ranger balloon and a 3.5/15 mm Multi-Link stent premounted on a high-pressure balloon were used to dilate the vessel (Fig. CC3–2). We did not use adjunctive abciximab, although in some laboratories this approach would not be inappropriate. The patient was discharged home the next day, and was given aspirin and ticlopidine; she was asymptomatic at 6-month follow-up.

Clinical Case 4. Angulated Vessel

A 50-year-old mailman has had crescendo angina for 5 months. He has been receiving maximum medical treatment for his angina, without any significant relief; he undergoes a diagnostic left heart catheterization, which shows a severe angulated lesion in a moderate size (estimated diameter 2.5 mm) diagonal branch (Fig. CC4–1). He does not have any other significant disease in the other coronary arteries, and his left ventricular function is normal.

An extra-support wire was used initially, but it created a subintimal dissection with acute closure (Fig. CC4–2). Therefore, a softer, floppy wire is now used instead; this wire is successfully placed in the distal vessel and the lesion is dilated with a 2.5 mm Ranger balloon at 6 atm. Flow is restored (Fig. CC4–3); a type C dissection is evident. The floppy wire is exchanged for an extra-support wire to straighten the vessel, and a 2.5/20 mm Gianturco-Roubin stent is successfully delivered (Fig. CC4–4).

Discussion: The angulation of coronary arteries is associated with reduced procedural success and high rate complication, es-

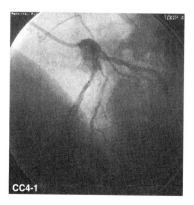
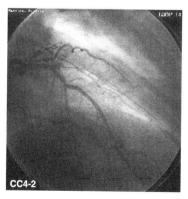

CC4-1   CC4-2

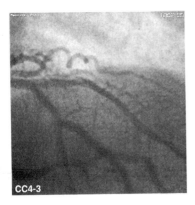
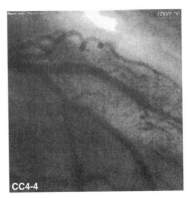

pecially acute closure secondary to dissection. The restenosis rate is increased as well.

The conventional 0.014″ wire is usually helpful to cross the lesion; a stiffer wire can be used if necessary (to straighten the vessel in order to allow the placement of a stent).

Use of noncompliant and long balloons was advocated, but recent data show that there is no difference between compliant and noncompliant balloons in terms of lumen enlargement and complication rates.

The atherectomy devices are generally contraindicated in severely angulated lesions, due to high risk of dissection or perforation.

When high-grade dissections appear in severely angulated lesions, coil stents can be more easily placed than slotted tubular stents.

If the attempts to dilate the angulated stenosis fail, bypass surgery should be considered if the vessel supplies a large area of myocardium. For vessels that supply smaller myocardial territories, such as in the case presented above, medical therapy would have been the best option.

Clinical Case 5. In-stent Restenosis

A 75-year-old woman underwent PTCA/stent (3.0×25 mm Multi-Link) of the proximal LAD 2 months ago; repeat angiogram (Fig.

CC5–1) reveals in-stent restenosis. What is the best treatment strategy?

Discussion: All of the following are currently acceptable:

- Rotational atherectomy
- DCA
- Balloon angioplasty
- Stent "sandwich"
- ELCA

In-stent restenosis is a "new" disease; since its pathogenesis is mostly intimal hyperplasia, debulking therapy has been advocated, especially if the process involves the whole stent. However, there are not enough data that clearly demonstrate superiority of one therapy over the others. With the use of IVUS, researchers have shown that PTCA improves the lumen by tissue extrusion out of the stent and by additional stent expansion in equal proportions. However, none of these techniques recover the lumen dimensions achieved during the initial stent implantation. The restenosis rate has been disappointingly high (clinical restenosis has ranged from 14% to 50%, depending on the type of lesion— longer lesions having higher restenosis rates).

PTCA appears to be adequate for focal lesions. Debulking therapy results in higher MLD, especially if it is followed by PTCA. However, this has not been translated into better clinical long-term results (target vessel revascularization and major adverse cardiac events).

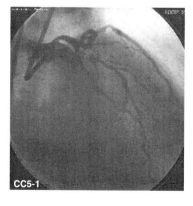
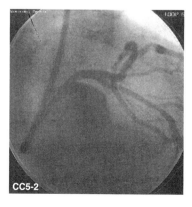

Diffuse lesions are perhaps better treated with debulking: DCA if the vessel is greater than 3.5 mm and rotational atherectomy for smaller vessels. Additionally, if IVUS is performed and reveals underexpansion of the stent, a larger balloon should be used as adjunctive therapy.

Brachytherapy appears promising. Short-term experience with β and γ radiation evaluated in small studies suggests that this technology is effective in reducing restenosis.

In this particular case, we performed balloon angioplasty alone using a 3.25 mm Quantum Ranger balloon (Fig. CC5–2).

Clinical Case 6. Intracoronary Thrombus

An 81-year-old male presents with a small non Q wave MI. He had undergone CABG 11 years earlier, receiving LIMA-LAD and 2 separate SVGs to the posterior descending coronary artery (PDA) and the first obtuse marginal branch. Angiogram of the SVG-OM reveals extensive thrombus in the distal body of the graft (Fig. CC6–1). The LIMA and SVG-PDA are patent. How would you approach this lesion?

Discussion: Appropriate therapy includes:

- TEC
- AngioJet® (Possis Medical, Inc., Minneapolis, MN) followed by PTCA
- Abciximab and PTCA
- Abciximab and staged PTCA to a later date
- Local infusion of thrombolytic

Large thrombus burden in an SVG has been associated with the no reflow phenomenon, as well as subsequent ischemia and MI if it cannot be reversed promptly.

Local delivery of thrombolytics is associated with bleeding complications, and the results have been inconsistent.

Alternatively, TEC has been used and is the only approved device in this setting. Its use is limited by bulkiness and cumbersome set

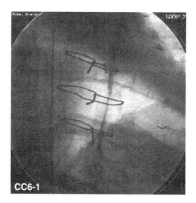

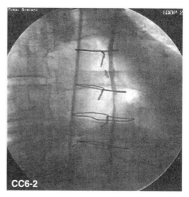

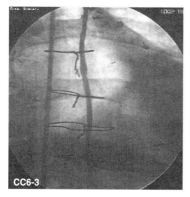

up. In addition, the clinical data supporting TEC atherectomy are weak. The availability of antiplatelet therapy and stents for the revascularization of these lesions has improved the primary success rate. The therapeutic approach of thrombotic SVG lesions continues to be a problem. New devices are being tested.

Reports presented at the ACC 47th Annual Scientific Sessions support the use of antiplatelet aggregation-receptor antagonists prior to interventional procedures; patients receiving Gp IIb/IIIa inhibitors prior to percutaneous revascularization have better outcomes.

This patient was treated with the standard dose of abciximab followed by I.V. heparin for 2 days, at which time angiogram was repeated (Fig. CC6–2). Significant reduction in thrombus burden was seen. The lesion was dilated and stented using a Multi-Link

3.75/15 mm stent. Transient no reflow was observed and re-sponded promptly to I.C. verapamil. The final result is seen in Fig-ure CC6–3.

Clinical Case 7. Ulceration and Thrombus

A 60-year-old firefighter develops exercise angina. The angiography shows a severely ulcerated lesion with haziness suggestive of throm-bus with TIMI 1–2 distal flow in a large (vessel diameter 3.6 mm) dominant RCA (Fig. CC7–1). The other vessels are free of significant disease; there are grade II collaterals from the LAD to the RCA.

The presence of plaque ulceration and superimposed thrombus prompt the use of abciximab.

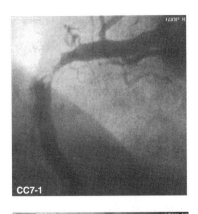
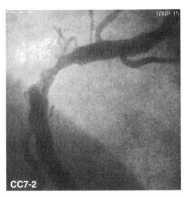
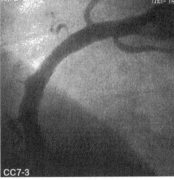

A Sport wire (Guidant/ACS Inc., Santa Clara, CA) is placed successfully in the distal vessel; a 3.5/15 mm Ranger balloon dilating catheter is used to predilate the stenosis. After two inflations the TIMI 3 flow is reestablished and patient is angina-free (Fig. CC7–2). A biliary stent PS 154M (Cordis, Johnson & Johnson, New Brunswick, NJ) is mounted on a 4.5/20 mm Mega Titan balloon (Cordis), but the attempts to advance the stent/balloon catheter are unsuccessful; hence, a premounted stent is used (4.0/15 mm Crown stent). The stent is successfully placed at the site of the stenosis; the balloon bursts at 12 atm. The 4.5 Mega Titan balloon is therefore placed inside the stent, but it bursts as well at 10 to 11 atm. Other balloons are tried for poststent high-pressure dilatation, but all burst at 10 to 12 atm. Final angiogram (Fig. CC7–3) shows an acceptable result, with +5% residual stenosis, no dissection, and TIMI 3 grade distal flow. The patient is discharged the next day on aspirin and ticlopidine. He has a negative nuclear imaging study at 4-month follow-up.

Discussion: Ulcerated lesions, consisting of flap of intimal tissue or fibrous plaque protruding into the lumen, have a negative effect on procedural outcome. A higher risk of acute closure, distal embolization, and no reflow must be anticipated. Some authors recommend use of I.V. heparin for 24 to 48 hours before intervention; others recommend I.C. lytic therapy. Systemic lytic therapy might be associated with increased risk of medial hemorrhage resulting in higher degrees of stenosis. With advent of Gp IIb/IIIa receptor blockers, the majority of laboratories would use abciximab.

The ideal mechanical treatment of thrombus is unknown. According to the results of the TOPIT trial, TEC may result in a lower incidence of non Q wave MI when compared to PTCA. The AngioJet rheolytic thrombectomy catheter is being evaluated in preliminary trials.

Although the initial teaching was that stenting is contraindicated in thrombus-reach lesions, recent advances in stent implantation, high-pressure deployment, and aggressive antiplatelet therapy resulted in marked decreases in thrombotic occlusions after stent implantation. The rate of subacute thrombosis in stented infarct vessels is 0% to 3%. The general opinion is that in the clinical setting of acute coronary syndromes, the association of thrombus does not result in adverse consequences from stenting. Heparin-coated stents are available in Europe.

Insertion of stents into small vessels with diameters less than 2.5 mm has been associated with high risk of acute closure and high mortality.

In our specific case, the presence of an ulcerated lesion increases the risk of acute closure with PTCA alone, and stenting is recommended.

Ionic contrast media offer an advantage over nonionic contrast media in reducing thrombus propagation.

The use of aspirin and ticlopidine upon discharge is the norm. Coumadin has not been shown to be beneficial.

Clinical Case 8. Revascularization in the Setting of Acute MI

A 46-year-old high school teacher presents with an inferior wall MI of 3 hours duration. Angiography (Fig. CC8–1) reveals a total occlusion of a dominant RCA (reference diameter 3.4 mm). The other vessels are free of disease. Patient is hemodynamically stable.

We used ionic low osmolar contrast. Abciximab was administered as bolus followed by I.V. drip. The occlusion was crossed with a high-torque floppy wire, and a 3.0 mm compliant balloon inflated at the lesion site reestablished flow. A 3.5/25 mm Multi-Link stent was placed at the site of the stenosis and was successfully deployed. Poststent high-pressure dilatation was performed using a 3.75/15 mm Quantum Ranger balloon (Fig. CC8–2).

Discussion: The following are different angioplasty approaches for acute MI: primary PTCA (PTCA without thrombolytic therapy), rescue PTCA (PTCA after failed lytic therapy), immediate PTCA (performed immediately after successful thrombolytic ther-

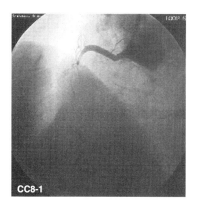
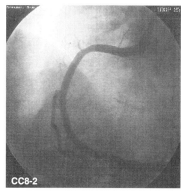

apy), and delayed PTCA (performed 1 to 7 days after thrombolytic therapy).

Primary PTCA should be strongly considered in high-risk patients: anterior MI, age greater than 70, HR greater than 100, BP less than 100 mm Hg, Killip class greater than 1.

In thrombolytic-eligible patients, primary PTCA reduces recurrent ischemia, reinfarction, length of hospital stay, and cost.

Primary PTCA results in acute patency of the infarcted vessel of 83% to 97% and in-hospital mortality of 1.5% to 9.3%.

Registry experience as well as randomized trials showed better results with PTCA versus thrombolytic therapy (higher procedural success, less stroke rate, and recurrent ischemia).

Important technical aspects to take into account in primary PTCA are:

- Use of ionic contrast material is indicated, due to less likelihood of thrombus formation; low osmolar agent is better, given its favorable hemodynamic profile.
- Start with a steerable, floppy wire and then "dotter" the lesion with the balloon catheter. Rapid reperfusion may increase the risk of reperfusion arrhythmias, especially in RCA lesions. Hypotension and bradycardia related to Bezold-Jarisch reflex can be anticipated with recanalization of totally occluded proximal RCA.

- After some antegrade flow is reestablished, the vessel distal to the occlusion should be sized and the operator should make sure that the wire is not in a small side branch.
- If after a long inflation at nominal size the result is sub-optimal (more than 30% residual stenosis or dissection is present), stenting is performed to decrease the risk of recurrent ischemia.
- The adjunctive pharmacologic therapy should include aspirin, ticlopidine, abciximab (if there is a large thrombus burden), I.C. nitroglycerin for spasm, and I.C. verapamil for "slow flow."

Clinical Case 9. SVG Disease. No Reflow Phenomenon

A 65-year-old recently retired male teacher with history of CABG 8 years ago develops angina while on a hiking trip. He has a positive exercise stress test. Coronary angiography reveals a patent LIMA to LAD and a patent vein graft to a large obtuse marginal branch. The native RCA is totally occluded proximally and the vein graft to distal RCA has moderate degeneration in the body of the graft (Fig. CC9–1).

What would be the best therapeutic choice?
  a. Repeat CABG
  b. Percutaneous revascularization
  c. Medical treatment

The operator proceeded with percutaneous revascularization. After a Sport wire was placed in the distal RCA via the vein graft, the lesion was dilated with a 3.0/15 Quantum Ranger balloon at 8 atm. Figure CC9–2 shows the angiography after the first inflation.

What would you do next?
  a. I.C. nitroglycerin
  b. I.C. abciximab
  c. I.C. verapamil

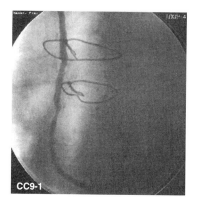

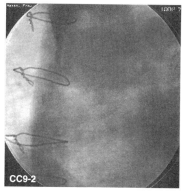

Two hundred micrograms of verapamil were given I.C. (Fig. CC9–3). The patient had already been receiving abciximab since the beginning of the case. What would you do next?

   a. Give more verapamil
   b. Implant a stent
   c. Use prolonged perfusion balloon inflation

A 3.5/30 Microstent was deployed (Fig. CC9–4). The patient returned after 3 months for a Viagra (Pfizer, New York, NY) prescription.

Discussion: This is a situation in which the other grafts are patent and therefore repeat CABG is not indicated.

Medical therapy involves the risk of vein graft occlusion, MI, and exercise angina, with decreased quality of life in a highly active person.

Percutaneous intervention is a good choice, although it is not risk free; risks include distal embolization, no reflow, restenosis, and MI.

In degenerated vein grafts the most important complication is no reflow. It complicates ~15% of degenerated vein graft interventions and frequently leads to MI and/or death; it cannot be treated with stents or CABG. The etiology of no reflow is distal embolization and microvascular spasm. Calcium channel blockers given I.C. reverse 65% of no reflow; to minimize the risk of

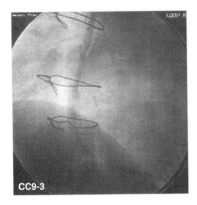
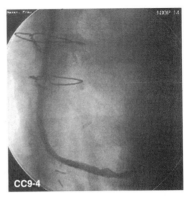

no reflow, verapamil may be given on a prophylactic basis. A temporary pacemaker should be inserted for interventions on degenerated vein grafts to RCA or dominant LCX, since no reflow in these situations is frequently associated with bradycardia and hypotension. Although sensibly less frequent, the no reflow phenomenon cannot be avoided even by using extraction devices such as TEC.

Thrombectomy with the AngioJet and Hydrolyzer are more useful for removing fresh thrombi than organized adherent thrombus specific to old vein grafts.

Covered stents (synthetic or natural) are being evaluated for degenerated vein graft treatment.

Clinical Case 10. LIMA Angioplasty

A 55-year-old farmer presents with unstable angina 5 years after CABG. The angiography shows two patent vein grafts to RCA and LCX and a 80% stenosis at the anastomotic site of LIMA to LAD (Fig. CC10–1).

To approach this lesion we used an 8F IMA guiding catheter from which 15 cm were cut at the proximal end; the hub was replaced

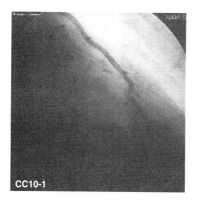 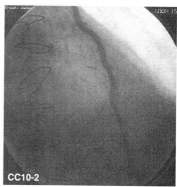

with an 8F introducer. The lesion was crossed with a long Hitorque intermediate wire and dilated with a 3.0 14K balloon dilating catheter. A 3.0/9 GFX stent was successfully placed (Fig. CC10–2). The patient was discharged the next day, taking aspirin and ticlopidine.

The following technical factors should be considered when treating IMA angioplasty:

- If the subclavian artery is very tortuous, the 60° LAO projection will elongate the aortic arch, allowing good visualization of the great vessels. If the subclavian artery is too tortuous, the ipsilateral brachial artery approach should be tried.
- IMA is prone to dissection and spasm and, therefore, pretreatment with nitroglycerin and/or verapamil is advised.
- Due to extreme length and tortuosity of this type of graft, we recommend use of low-profile balloons and long shaft (150 cm) balloons or short guiding catheters (90 cm).
- When stenting any severe lesion at the distal anastomotic site, one potential problem is the size mismatching between the graft and the native vessel. In this case it is important to taper the stent with appropriately sized balloons so that the correctly deployed and dilated stent will have a funnel-shaped configuration.

Clinical Case 11. Spiral Dissection and Abrupt Closure

A 58-year-old male accountant was admitted for elective percutaneous revascularization of a 90% eccentric stenosis of mid LAD (vessel diameter 3.7 mm). Previous angiography showed a 60% lesion in mid RCA and a 75% lesion in a large obtuse marginal branch. There was no collateral circulation. The left ventricular function was within normal limits.

The lesion was crossed with a Sport wire without difficulty. A 4.0/15 Quantum Ranger balloon was inflated to 6 atm at the site of the stenosis. This resulted in a suboptimal result, with ≥30% residual stenosis and a local complex dissection with TIMI 2 distal flow. Abciximab was started. Patient had anginal pain and ST segment elevation on ECG. Rapid stabilization of the dissection was tried by attempting the placement of a stent. None of the stents used would cross the lesion (Multi-Link, GFX, Crown, Gianturco Roubin II). The attempt to place a long Lifestream perfusion balloon (St. Jude Medical, Sylmar, CA) was unsuccessful as well. An exchange catheter was placed in the distal vessel in the attempt to exchange the Sport wire for a 0.014″ Platinum-Plus wire (Boston Scientific/SciMed Inc.). During the wire exchange, the wire position was inadvertently lost (Fig. CC11–1) and further attempts to recross the lesion resulted in a spiral dissection with abrupt closure (Fig. CC11–2). An intra-aortic balloon pump was inserted and the patient underwent emergency CABG. He was discharged home after 1 week, stable. The peak CPK was 350 and there were no Q waves in anterior leads. Follow-up ECHO at 4 months showed normal left ventricular function.

Discussion:

- It is possible that the 4.0 mm balloon was oversized and that the inflation resulted in a dissection.
- Once the wire position is lost, further attempts to recross should be made with very flexible wires (eg, Hitorque floppy), and not with extra-support wires.
- Unless there is a contraindication, such a patient should be sent to emergency surgery with a long perfusion balloon in place to maintain distal perfusion. An intra-aortic balloon pump should be inserted as soon as possible.

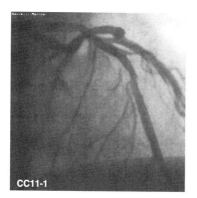 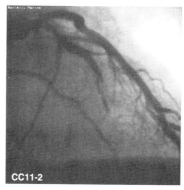

- Obviously, maintaining guidewire access to the distal vessel is of paramount importance; loss of the wire position may have catastrophic consequences.

Clinical Case 12. Coronary Aneurysm

A 62-year-old housewife presents with unstable angina and new inferior wall T wave inversions, 1 year after placement of two Palmaz-Schatz stents in the mid RCA. The angiography reveals an isolated severe stenosis in the middle of a fusiform aneurysmal dilatation 4.0 mm in diameter, possibly in an area where the two previous stents did not overlap (Fig. CC12–1). There is a 60% RCA ostial stenosis as well. The stenosis was crossed without difficulty, using a Choice PT wire; the lesion was dilated with a Quantum Ranger 3.5 mm balloon; abciximab was used. Figure CC12–2 shows the final result. The patient was discharged home on 325 mg of aspirin daily and she was asymptomatic at 3-month follow-up.

Discussion:

- The Coronary Artery Surgery Study (CASS) defined coronary aneurysm as an arterial dilatation that exceeds 1.5 times the diameter of the normal adjacent vessel.
- The incidence after angioplasty is 4% to 7%, and 10% after atherectomy.
- It was hypothesized that as coronary arteries move and the stent is immobile, sheer forces would concentrate

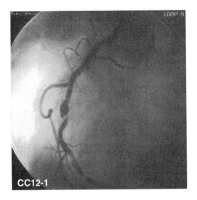
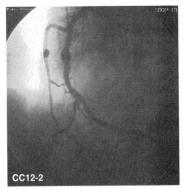

at the interface between the intima and the stent edges; this will interfere with healing process and will result in gradual wall thinning, weakening, and aneurysm formation by 32 weeks post stent implant.

- The coronary aneurysms related to percutaneous revascularization procedures are divided into two types: early and late. The early aneurysm is recognized during or soon after the procedure and represents pseudoaneurysm (contained perforation), which poses a high risk of rupture. Late-developing aneurysm, such as the one presented in our case, remains asymptomatic.
- The question of stenting such a lesion does not have an unanimous answer; if a stent is placed at the site of the dilated stenosis, high-pressure stent dilation should be performed with tapered and short balloons in order to fully expand the stent inside the aneurysm but not to over dilate the unaffected vessel.
- IVUS is useful for assessing the extent and nature of coronary aneurysms.

Clinical Case 13. Coronary Spasm

A 40-year-old man undergoes a treadmill stress test for atypical chest pain. He exercises 8 minutes Bruce protocol and stops because of leg fatigue. Two minutes into the recovery, he starts to have chest pain and ST segment elevation in inferior leads, associated with second-degree AV block and hypotension. Fluid resuscitation is performed and low-dose nitroglycerin is started. He is brought emergently to cardiac catheterization laboratory; the angiography reveals a significant stenosis in proximal-mid RCA with TIMI 1 distal flow (Fig. CC13–1). A superimposed coronary spasm is suspected and 200 μg of nitroglycerin is given I.C. Shortly after, the patient admits that the chest pain is much improved. Repeat angiography reveals mild nonobstructive disease with a maximum stenosis of 20% in mid-distal RCA and TIMI 3 grade distal flow (Fig. CC13–2). Patient is started on verapamil and discharged home symptom-free; he is angina-free at 1-month follow-up, when a maximal stress test is also negative for symptoms or ECG changes.

Discussion:

- Spontaneous coronary artery spasm is the very unpredictable substrate of Prinzmetal's angina. The arterial spasm occurs more frequently at the site of moderate or severe fixed stenoses, but also could be seen in mildly diseased or normal arteries.
- Medical management with calcium channel blockers is the treatment of choice.
- Coronary stenting and even CABG are used for patients who fail medical treatment; the restenosis rate is higher and postoperative MI early graft closure and recurrent angina are more frequent.

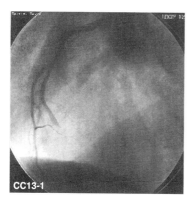

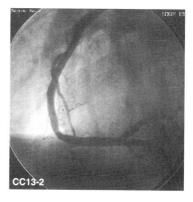

Clinical Case 14. Long Lesion

A 72-year-old hospital volunteer presents with exertional angina that she has had for approximately 4 months. She is currently on maximum medical treatment. In the last week, the patient has had two resting angina episodes, relieved with S.L. nitroglycerin. Coronary angiography (Fig. CC14–1) reveals a long stenosis in mid LAD (reference vessel 3.0 mm). The RCA and circumflex are free of significant disease. There are no collaterals. Left ventricular function is normal.

Issues to consider:

I. Clinical
    indications
    alternative treatments available
    risk
    prognosis

II. Technical
    which guider
    which wire
    debulking necessary?
    stent versus plain old balloon angioplasty (POBA)
    complications
    pharmacologic adjunctive therapy

Discussion:

1. The patient has unstable angina due to a long, type C, mid-LAD lesion. This lesion must be treated. The alternatives include medical treatment, percutaneous revascularization, and CABG. No study has shown a survival benefit or decrease in the rate of MI for CABG over medical treatment for patients with single vessel disease. This patient, however, is symptomatic and already on maximum medical treatment; therefore she needs revascularization.

The objectives of coronary revascularization in patients with single vessel disease are the alleviation of symptoms or ischemia; no trials have shown a survival advantage of surgery.

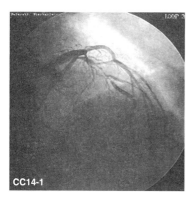 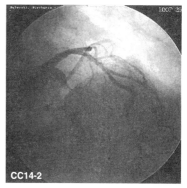

2. There is an inverse relationship between the angioplasty success and the lesion length. Some studies
have shown that there is an increased rate of complications related to lesion length. The restenosis rate is
increased.

In this long lesion, rotablation is preferred.

The burr selection is guided by the treated vessel dimension; the
maximal burr size should be 60% to 80% of the reference vessel
diameter. The initial burr size should be at least 0.5 mm less than
maximal burr suitable for the case.

The guider catheter should be chosen according to the final burr
diameter: burrs ≤2.0 mm can be accommodated by giant-lumen
8F guide; 2.38 mm burr can be advanced through a giant-lumen
9F guide; for 2.50 mm burrs a 10F guide is necessary.

In our specific case, an 8F guider with side holes was used. It is
believed that the side holes help to improve the particle clearance
during the procedure. Because the vessel is straight, an Extra-
Support wire was used. An initial 1.75 mm burr successfully
crossed the lesion, followed by 2.0 mm and 2.25 mm burrs. Short
20- to 30-second runs were used.

Adjunctive PTCA was performed using a low-pressure inflation
with slightly oversized long balloon.

The second diagonal branch was dilated using a 2.5 mm ACE balloon, without any complication.

Due to the clinical presentation (unstable coronary syndrome) and suspicion of thrombus on angiography, abciximab was used.

The final result is shown in Figure CC14–2. The patient was discharged home 48 hours later. She returned with unstable angina due to focal restenosis of mid LAD. After PTCA, a stent was placed. If the patient comes back with restenosis, she will be referred for surgical revascularization.

Clinical Case 15. Coronary Dissection After Rotablation

A 40-year-old nurse is admitted for elective percutaneous revascularization. He has had stable angina for the last 2 months; he is on daily aspirin but he refuses to take antianginal medication. His angiography (Fig. CC15–1) reveals a 15-mm-long 90% stenosis in mid RCA (vessel diameter 3.0 mm); left ventricular function is normal.

Because of the length of the lesion, rotablation revascularization technique is used. A 1.5 mm burr is used first, followed by a 2.25 mm burr. One 40-second run is performed with this burr; during this run the rpm drops from 160,000 rpm to a minimum of

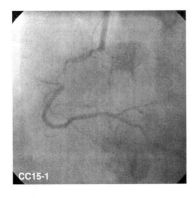
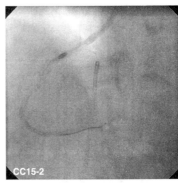

CC15-1   CC15-2

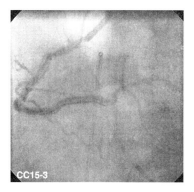

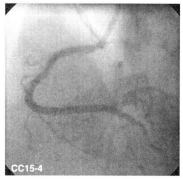

150,000 rpm. The patient starts to have chest pain. The burr is withdrawn and angiography shows a spiral dissection (Figs. CC15–2 and CC15–3). This is treated with a balloon inflation (Lifestream 3.25/20 mm) at low pressure, followed by placement of a Multi-Link 3.0/25 mm stent. The final result is shown in Figure CC15–4.

Discussion: The dissection postrotablation technique occurs usually within the calcified plaque extending to the noncalcified vessel wall after PTCA.

The possible mechanisms of rotablation-induced dissections are:

- Inappropriate step-burr sizing; a gradual increase in the burr size is recommended. In the case presented above, a more gradual approach using a second 1.75 mm or a 2.0 mm burr would have been indicated.
- Presence of moderate or severe angulation. One such typical case would be the ostium of a severely angulated circumflex.
- Burr deceleration by more than 5000 RPM.
- Long runs (usually ≥30 seconds).

In case of dissection, the use of slightly oversized balloon inflation at low pressure may be beneficial. If the dissection persists, stent deployment is recommended to cover the dissected portion of the vessel.

Clinical Case 16. Multivessel PTCA

A 50-year-old retired veteran presents with chronic stable angina, and is on maximal medical treatment. He has been diabetic for 20 years. A stress test reveals anterior and lateral wall ischemia. The angiography is performed, and two significant lesions are found in the LAD and circumflex (Fig. CC16–1); there are collaterals from circumflex to distal LAD; RCA has a 50% to 75% lesion in mid vessel; the left ventricular function is normal. The patient does not have a patent LIMA, due to a thoracic trauma during the war.

Questions:

1.   What revascularization procedure serves him better: CABG or multivessel PTCA?

2.   Is the lack of LIMA conduit important in your decision?

3.   Is the patient's lifestyle an important component in the therapeutic approach?

4.   If you proceed with percutaneous revascularization, in what order would you approach these lesions?

5.   Would you dilate all lesions at the same time or prefer a staged procedure?

6.   Is the involvement of the first septal perforator branch of any importance in your decision?

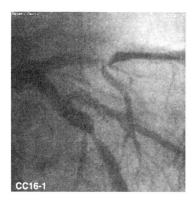
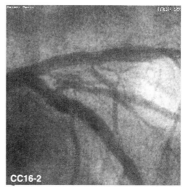

CC16-1

CC16-2

Discussion:

1. and 2.   Generally, CABG is recommended in 3-vessel disease, LM disease, multivessel disease with reduced left ventricular function, extensive disease, and diabetes mellitus (with the provision of using internal artery mammary conduit to LAD).

Multivessel PTCA is recommended for 2-vessel disease with preserved left ventricular function, suitable anatomy, and salvage procedure (not candidates for CABG). The presence of cerebrovascular disease, COPD, and younger age usually favors a percutaneous approach.

In the BARI and CABRI trials, patients with multivessel disease and treated diabetes mellitus had lower cardiac mortality if treated with CABG. The difference was made by the use of IMA conduit. If only SVGs were used, the outcomes were comparable.

3. The patient's wish to minimize the number of reinterventions (8% for CABG and 54% for PTCA) and daily medicines favors the surgical approach.
4. From a technical standpoint, the vessel with better collaterals should be dilated first. If there are no collaterals, start with the vessel serving an area with more severe ischemia.
5. Some authors support the "next-day" staging strat-

egy, in which patients are revascularized during their first hospitalization. This is a comfortable, cost-effective approach that should be used if the original result is optimal at the next day angiography. If the result became suboptimal, the vessel should be optimally dilated and the rest of the lesions treated in a few weeks.

6. The presence of the septal perforator branch does not interfere in any way with the treatment of the parent vessel.

In the case presented above, the patient underwent multiple PTCA. The LAD lesion was dilated first with use a Quantum Ranger 3.0/15 mm balloon inflated twice at 6 atm and followed by placement of a Crown 3.0/22 mm stent. Next, the circumflex artery was dilated using the same balloon, followed by placement of a Multi-Link 3.5/15 mm stent. Abciximab infusion was used. The result is shown in Figure CC16–2.

The patient was discharged home the next day and a stress test 2 months later revealed mild ischemia of the inferior wall. The angiography revealed widely patent LAD and circumflex and a 50% to 75% lesion in the RCA. Completeness of revascularization is of prognostic importance and therefore we opted for balloon dilatation and stent placement.

Clinical Case 17. Perforation

An 80-year-old woman is admitted with unstable angina and ischemic changes in inferior leads. She had a CABG 10 years ago. The angiography reveals patent LIMA to LAD, patent SVG to circumflex, and a severe stenosis of the anastomosis of SVG to distal RCA (reference vessel 3.0 mm). The lesion (Fig. CC17–1) is successfully dilated with use of an extra-support guidewire, a compliant 3.5/15 mm balloon, and a Wiktor stent 3.0/15 mm deployed at 12 atm (balloon ruptures after 30 seconds of inflation). Final angiography shows a good result but a contained perforation as seen in Figure CC17–2.

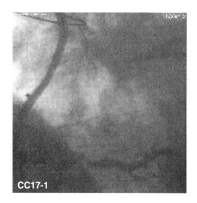 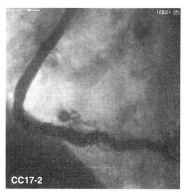

Questions to consider:

1.   What are the potential causes of this perforation?

2.   What should be done next?

3.   Is this patient at high risk of cardiac tamponade?

Discussion:

1. The patient's characteristics (elderly woman) put her in a higher risk group for perforation. The potential reasons for this event include use of an oversized balloon (balloon:artery ratio ≥1.2), balloon rupture, and use of stiff guidewire for stent delivery.
2. Assess the hemodynamic stability of the patient; notify the cardiac surgeons and the operating room; place a perfusion balloon (balloon:artery ratio = 1.0) at the site of perforation and inflate for 10 to 15 minutes. If after the first inflation the perforation is still present, inflate the balloon for additional time (15 to 30 minutes). Do not forget to intermittently flush the

central lumen with heparinized saline to prevent clotting. Do not administer additional heparin. If there is a stable intervention result and no further dye extravasation, the patient should be admitted to an intensive care setting and observed for 36 to 48 hours. This is contained perforation. Reversal of heparin effect with protamine is necessary in cases of perforation resulting in jet extravasation or cavity spilling. Usually, serial ECHOs are recommended every 6 to 12 hours to assess for continuous bleeding. If stable, the patient can be discharged on aspirin and ticlopidine.

3. Cardiac tamponade is unusual after CABG. Intramuscular or mediastinal hemorrhage can be seen.

Clinical Case 18. Tortuous Vessel

A 75-year-old man is admitted for elective revascularization of a severe stenosis of the distal RCA (vessel diameter 3.0 mm) (Fig. CC18–1). He has unstable angina and needs colon surgery for an invasive colon cancer.

Questions to consider:

1.   Is this a high-risk procedure?

2.   What equipment do you have in mind?

Discussion:

1. This is a tortuous vessel. Therefore, there is a higher possibility of procedural failure due to inability to reach the lesion (cross with the guidewire, reach with the balloon, place a stent if dissection occurs). In cases of proximal vessel tortuosity, deep seating of the guider catheter is recommended; in this case the op-

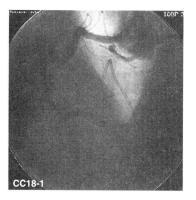

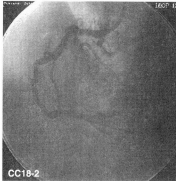

erator has to manipulate the guider catheter ex-
tremely carefully because of the immediate proximity
of an anomalous circumflex take off.
2. We used a long, 30 cm arterial sheath; this will make
the manipulation of the guiding catheter easier in the
case of iliac artery tortuosity.

The guider catheter used in this case was an 8F hockey stick-
shaped guider catheter, because of the horizontal take off.

We opted for a Choice PT wire; this successfully crossed the proximal vessel tortuosities as well as the lesion itself.

A Quantum Ranger 3.0/15 mm balloon (Boston Scientific/SciMed
Inc.) was advanced close to the lesion but could not be placed at
the lesion site. An exchange catheter was used to replace the
Choice PT with a stiffer wire (Platinum-Plus). The same balloon
was tried again, unsuccessfully. Finally, a 14K 2.0 was placed at
the site of the stenosis and inflated at 6 atm for 30 seconds. This
resulted in a suboptimal result. Therefore, the NC Ranger was
placed successfully at the site of the stenosis, and inflated at 6 atm
for 30 seconds, three times, until the result was considered optimal
(Fig. CC18–2). An attempt to place a stent was not made because of
anticipated difficulty and because the result was "stent like."

In negotiating tortuous vessels, do not forget the following:

• long femoral sheaths may ease the manipulation of the
guider;

- choose a guider that aligns well, offers a stable position, and good "back-up support";
- if unsuccessful, the alternatives include "deep-seating" the guider, using a larger diameter guider, or using the brachial approach;
- over-the-wire balloons are more trackable than monorail;
- if stenting is necessary, use coiled wire designs; they are more trackable.

Clinical Case 19. Protected Left Main

A 72-year-old male has developed class III angina (CCSC) over the last 6 months. He had previously received (12 years ago) 3-vessel coronary bypass grafting including LIMA to the LAD and separate vein grafts to the first obtuse marginal and the PDA.

Angiogram (Fig. CC19–1) revealed a patent LIMA and total occlusion of both vein grafts, the native RCA was also occluded and the LM had a high-grade lesion distally at the bifurcation. The LAD was occluded as well, and there were well developed (grade III) collaterals to the PDA, mostly from the LAD. Left ventricular function was normal.

Discussion: Revascularization strategies include the following:

- Redo bypass grafting: due to the presence of a well functioning LIMA graft, this will not be the initial strategy of choice despite the fact that it is able to accomplish complete revascularization.
- LM/circumflex revascularization: debulking would be preferably the first step. One could argue that IVUS might help make that decision, but it is unlikely that it will *change* that. Rotational atherectomy with 1.75 and 2.25 mm burrs was performed in this case. It was necessary to wire the lesion initially with a high-torque floppy wire and to exchange it with the help of a transfer catheter (a small balloon [2.0] can also be used) to a roto-floppy wire, the latter being a more difficult wire to torque and negotiate through the lesion. Subsequently, a 3.5×20 mm balloon was used

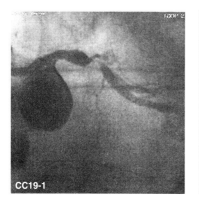

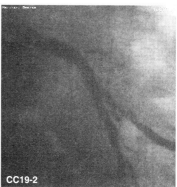

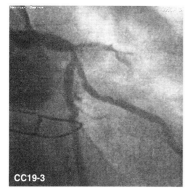

followed by the implantation of a 4.0×22 mm Crown stent (Figs. CC19–2 and CC19–3).

- Revascularization of the RCA was not attempted; neither on the native vessel, due to length and age of the occlusion (present at the time of the initial bypass), nor on the vein graft, as this was occluded at the aorto-ostial level signifying and old occlusion.

Clinical Case 20. Bifurcation Lesion

A 47-year-old male is referred for cardiac catheterization after he develops class II angina and has a positive nuclear stress test (myoview) for ischemia in the lateral wall at Bruce stage 2. Angiogram

(Fig. CC20–1) reveals a bifurcation lesion in the mid circumflex with a high-grade lesion in the marginal and totally occluded distal AV groove circumflex that fills retrograde via left-to-left collaterals.

Discussion: Bifurcational lesions are difficult to treat and have high restenosis rates. Debulking therapy might offer an advantage, as it decreases plaque shifting (snow plow effect). Stenting is problematic and initial enthusiasm with "T" or "Y" stenting has diminished due to high restenosis rates (up to 70%) that involve the bifurcation in up to 40% of the cases. In this particular case, there is no true main vessel-side branch approach (stent the main vessel and dilate across the stent the side branch). The lesion was double wired and initial PTCA (3.0×15) of the AVG-LCX (atri-

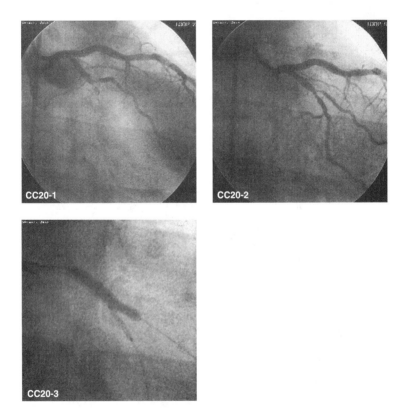

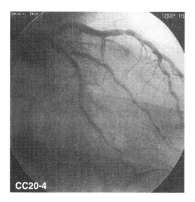
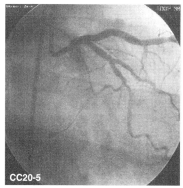

oventricular groove-left circumflex) was done (Fig. CC20–2), followed by "Y" stenting.

A 3.0×12 mm GFX stent was positioned in the AVG-LCX (distal to the bifurcation) and a balloon was inflated (low atm) in the proximal AVG-LCX and into the marginal; the stent was pulled back and deployed (Fig. CC20–3). Subsequently, a 3.0×9 mm GFX stent was advanced to the marginal with the proximal stent positioned in the AVG-LCX at the bifurcation, and deployed (Fig. CC20–4). The final angiogram is shown in Figure CC20–5.

Clinical Case 21. Spiral Dissection

A 65-year-old woman presenting with unstable angina and elevated troponin undergoes coronary angiogram that reveals a totally occluded RCA and well developed left-to-right collaterals (Figs. CC21–1 and CC21–2).

The lesion is crossed with a hydrophilic wire (Shinobi; Cordis, Johnson & Johnson) without difficulty; however, as the wire is advanced it becomes apparent that it has created a dissection plane

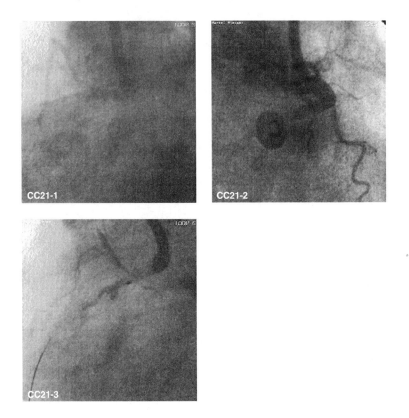

(Fig. CC21–3); the wire is withdrawn and the lesion recrossed. Following balloon inflation, antegrade flow is restored but an extensive dissection plane is noted in addition to reduced flow distally (Figs. CC21–4 and CC21–5).

Multiple stents are implanted starting at the distal RCA before the PDA, for a total of 4 (3.0×24 mm GFX, 3.0×12 mm GFX, and two 3.0×15 mm Multi-Link HP) (Figs. CC21–6 and CC21–7).

Discussion: Extensive dissection from the wire is a frightening situation, as it is possible that the true lumen can never be found. In this case it also jeopardized the collateral flow. Fortunately, with the availability of stents, these kind of problems rarely end up in the operating room, as long as wire access is maintained.

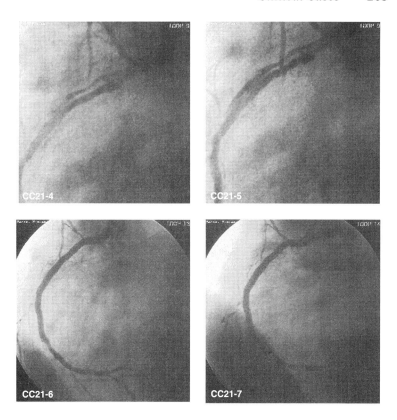

Clinical Case 22. Post-stent Dissection

A 47-year-old woman presents with an inferior wall MI that has been treated with thrombolytics at another hospital. She is transferred for coronary angiogram after an episode of resting angina the following day. Initial angiogram is shown (Fig. CC22–1). The lesion is crossed easily with a high-torque intermediate wire and balloon angioplasty, followed by deployment of a 4.0×22 mm Crown stent (Fig. CC22–2). A stepdown is noted at the distal edge of the stent.

After I.C. nitroglycerin was given and while preparation for IVUS evaluation was being set up, a second angiogram (Fig. CC22–3) revealed worsening of the lumen distal to the stent and associated reduced forward flow (TIMI 2) (Fig. CC22–4).

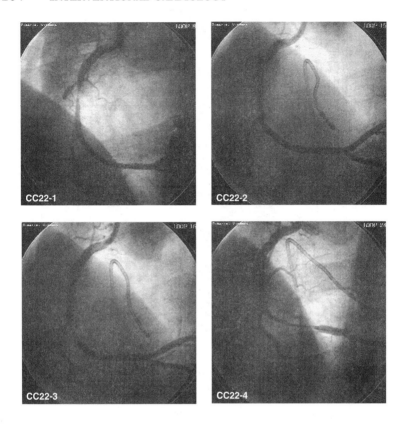

A 3.5×30 mm GFX stent was advanced through the Crown stent and deployed at the distal margin of the spiral dissection. Afterward, a proximal retrograde dissection was noted with abrupt closure (TIMI 0) (Fig. CC22–5) that required a 3.5×25 mm Multi-Link stent, restoring flow. Note the dissection outside the stent in the proximal RCA (Fig. CC22–6).

An area in between the Crown stent and the distal GFX is not covered with the stent. With difficulty, only a 9.0×35 mm GFX could be advanced to that location and deployed (Fig. CC22–7). Additionally, the proximally placed Multi-Link was post-dilated to 4.0 mm.

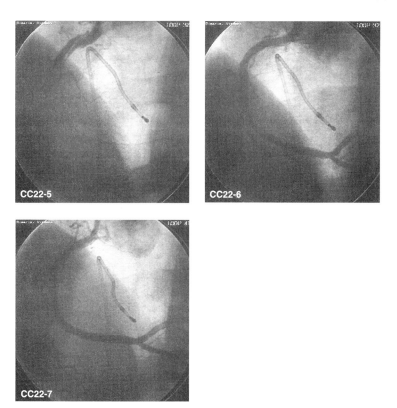

Discussion: Spiral stent edge dissections are rare but pose a challenge to the operator, as all of the distal stents must pass through the initially deployed stent; this increases the risk of stent migration. Newer self-expandable stents may be preferable; however, adequate guiding support and perhaps a softer wire that allows for less "wire bias" are essential. IVUS provides the operator with the opportunity to evaluate stent deployment in dubious situations. It is still to be determined whether routine use of IVUS will improve clinical outcomes during routine stent cases.

It has been suggested that a CFR greater than 0.94 is equivalent to optimal stent deployment by IVUS.

Clinical Case 23. Intravascular Ultrasound

Match each of the following IVUS images with its corresponding diagnosis.

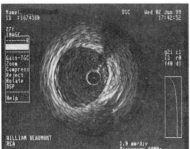

Image #1

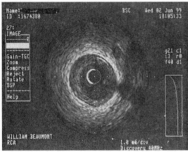

Image #2

Image #3

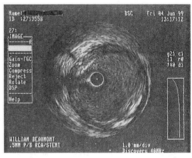

Image #4

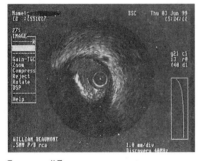

Image #5

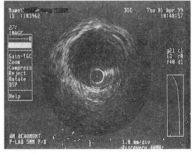

Image #6

a. Soft plaque
b. Flush
c. Fibrotic plaque
d. Calcium
e. Normal Vessel
f. Nonuniform rotational distortion (NURD)

ANSWERS: #1-e, #2-f, #3-a, #4-c, #5-d, #6-b

Discussion: *Normal vessel* morphology visualized by ultrasound comprises the following layers:

- Intima—the inner layer beneath which there is internal elastic lamina.
- Media—composed of multiple layers of smooth muscle cells; it has a mean thickness of 200 μm. Media is a sonolucent zone, less echodense than intima and adventitia due to lower collagen content. External elastic lamina encircles the media.
- Adventitia—composed of fibrous tissue, incorporating vasa vasorum, nerves, and lymphatics; its thickness ranges from 300 to 500 μm.

Distinct trilaminar appearance will be detected with IVUS in 50% of cases; the rest will appear monolayered.

NURD is an artefact of mechanical devices that results from excessive catheter bending. Another common artefact is "ring-down halo," which is caused by multiple oscillations around the catheter surface.

Plaque composition resulting in different echogenicity allowed the description of three different types of plaques:

- *soft or fatty plaque* is less echogenic than the adventitia;
- *fibrous plaque* has similar echogenicity to adventitia;
- *calcified plaque* is more echogenic than adventitia. It appears as a bright echo with shading behind, obscuring the deeper layers ("accoustic shadowing"). More than 180° of calcium is required to achieve a mass that is identifiable by angiography.

Match the following:

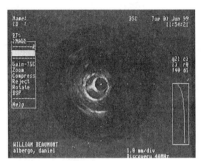
Image #7

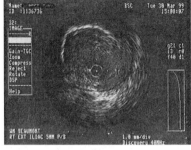
Image #8

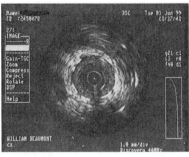
Image #9

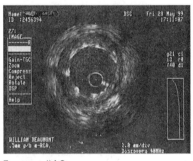
Image #10

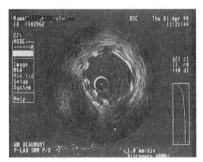
Image #11

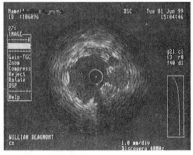
Image #12

a. In-stent restenosis
b. Guide
c. Underdeployed stent
d. Full stent aposition
e. Dissection

ANSWERS: #7-b, #8-e, #9-a, #10-c, #11-d, #12-c

Discussion: Coronary dissection can be detected with IVUS. Areas that are prone to dissection are:

- the thinnest portion of the plaque within an eccentric lesion
- regions of differing elasticity
- localized calcium

In-stent restenosis is characterized by neointimal hyperplasia, which appears as homogenous material. Therapeutic approaches to this new entity include balloon angioplasty using a larger, non-compliant balloon, rotablation atherectomy, and excimer laser angioplasty.

Complete apposition of the stent is expressed by:

- a symmetry index (ratio of stent minor diameter/major diameter) of greater than 0.7;
- a gap between the struts greater than 0.3 mm;
- CSA index of greater than 0.8; CSA index represents the ratio of minimal CSA of stent/CSA of normal reference vessel (average CSA proximal and distal to the stent).

Clinical Case 24. PTCA and Stent Implantation

The following images represent an optimal result after PTCA and stent implantation
a. True
b. False

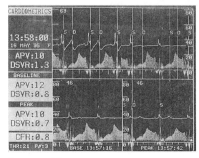

Image #1   Image #2

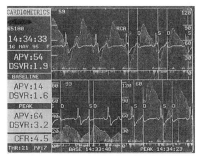

Image #3

ANSWER: a

The images represent an excellent response to PTCA and stent.

Velocity parameters displayed in the images represent:

- *Average peak velocity* should be greater than 20 cm/s in basal state and greater than 30 cm/s in hyperemic state;
- *diastolic/systolic mean velocity ratio* should be greater than 1.7 for LAD and greater than 1.4 for distal RCA;
- *proximal/distal mean velocity ratio* should be less than 1.7; this parameter is also known as *translesional velocity gradient;*
- *distal coronary flow reserve* should be greater than 2.0.

Abnormalities in microcirculation (Syndrome X, PTCA post acute MI, hypertension) may decrease CFR. Therefore, the ratio of distal hyperemic average peak velocity/mean aortic pressure (*fractional flow reserve*) is useful because it is independent of hemodynamic changes.

Chapter 9

Pearls

❦ Only one randomized trial (ACME) compared PTCA with medical therapy in patients with single vessel disease and stable angina, a positive stress test, or MI within the prior 3 months to PTCA or medical therapy:

✓ PTCA was more effective in relieving angina and improving performance on the treadmill.
✓ PTCA costs were higher.
✓ There was no significant difference in the rate of MI or death between the two groups.

❦ The benefits of CABG versus multivessel PTCA in the diabetic population are only seen in patients who have had a mammary artery bypass.

❦ There is no difference in death and acute MI at long-term follow-up between PTCA and CABG patients with multivessel disease, except for diabetic patients, who did better with CABG. The study did not include stent technique.

❦ The Evaluation of IIb/IIIa Platelet Inhibitor for Stenting (EPISTENT) trial showed that *stenting and abciximab* had the lowest composite endpoint (death, MI, TVR) at 6 months. Diabetic patients responded in a similar fashion.

❦ *Threatened vessel closure* is defined as a combination of ≥50% residual stenosis, severe dissection, angina, or ECG signs of ischemia. In this situation, stenting will reduce the death rate by 5%, and MI and CABG rates by 35%.

❦ Chronic total occlusions should be stented.

❦ Maximal coronary dilatation (up to 30%) is best obtained with an I.C. bolus of 100 μg to 300 μg of nitroglycerin; the peak effect is at 1 minute, and there are minimal systemic effects.

❦ Whenever possible, chose the end-diastolic frame for analysis: the kinetic flow is minimal and the vessel filling by contrast dye is optimal.

❦ *Angiographic restenosis:* ≥50% MLD at follow-up.

❦ *Acute gain:* immediate change in MLD resulting from the procedure.

❦ *Late loss:* the difference between follow-up MLD and immediate postprocedure MLD.

❦ *Loss index:* the slope of the regression line of late loss as a function of acute gain. Examples of loss indices: POBA, TEC—45/100; stent, DCA—50/100; and Roto—69/100.

❦ IVUS uses high frequency, resulting in greater resolution and lower depth (20 to 50 MHZ transducers/2.9F to 3.5F catheters).

❦ Heparin should be given for diagnostic IVUS imaging.

❦ Atherosclerotic plaques frequently accumulate at the bifurcations, where the blood turbulence is maximal.

❦ IVUS is very useful for appreciating the vasculopathy in transplant recipients who have a high rate of false-negative angiographies, because of the diffuse nature of the disease (concentric intimal thickening).

❦ Full apposition of the stent to the wall represents the most important IVUS criterion of adequate stent deployment.

❦ Symmetry index = MLD/maximal lumen diameter. It should be ≥70/100 (≥0.7).

❦ The correlation between sestamibi perfusion imaging and CFR measurement with Doppler guidewire is excellent.

❦ Up to 25% to 30% of people have a negative Allen test and are unsuitable for the radial artery approach.

❦ In primary lesions, the restenosis rate is higher for those with high cellularity in the fibrous plaque.

❦ Atherectomy does not result in better late angiographic or clinical outcomes in patients with lesions of the proximal LAD.

❦ With laser angioplasty, restenosis is due to thermal injury.

❦ Unstable angina is associated with white thrombus as shown by angioscopy.

❦ Transmyocardial revascularization is associated with improvement in symptoms, but does not improve heart function or survival.

❦ After PTCA, the restenosis occurs between 3 and 6 months; it is rare in the first month or after 12 months.

❦ Dissection post PTCA and deep cut after DCA do not increase the risk of restenosis.

❦ Unstable angina and diabetes are risk factors for restenosis.

❦ Ostial lesions, total occlusions, and long lesions increase the risk of restenosis.

❦ Residual stenosis ≥30% increases the risk of restenosis.

❦ There is high risk of thrombosis with biliary stents deployed in vessels with diameter ≤4 mm.

❦ IVUS criteria for optimal stent deployment include the following:

✓ CSA index ≥0.8
✓ good apposition
✓ symmetry index ≥0.7

❦ Acute MI is not a contraindication to stenting.

❦ The most common site of aortic atherosclerosis is the aortic bifurcation.

❦ Symptomatic carotid artery stenosis ≥60% and asymptomatic carotid artery stenosis ≥70% benefit from surgery.

❦ Claudication and an ABI of 0.6 to 0.9 signify single segment occlusion or well collateralized stenosis.

❦ Claudication and an ABI of 0.3 to 0.6 signify multiple segment disease.

❦ End-diastole absolute peak velocity ≥100 cm/s suggests severe stenosis.

❦ Flexible wires are less steerable; less flexibility offers more torque control.

❦ Side-branch protection is recommended for any side branch ≥2.0 mm in diameter with or without ostial stenosis originating from the parent vessel lesion.

❦ Stents offer an ~ 30% reduction in restenosis in de novo lesions compared with balloon angioplasty.

❦ Intrastent restenosis is IH.

❦ The prognosis of asymptomatic stent restenosis is excellent with medical treatment.

❦ Ionic contrast agents inhibit both platelet aggregation and coagulation when compared to nonionic agents.

❦ When the culprit vessel is not obvious in acute MI patients with multivessel disease, CABG is the best option.

❦ For bare stents, use a semicompliant or compliant balloon, so that the same balloon can be used for high-pressure inflations.

❦ When ostial lesions are dilated, use high-pressure, noncompliant balloons because of extra rigidity and tissue elasticity.

❦ For aorto-ostial lesions, use balloons that are long enough to prevent "watermelon seeding."

❦ If an aorto-ostial lesion does not fully expand despite high-pressure dilatation with noncompliant balloon, debulking is required.

❦ The proximal 2 mm of the stent should be flared against the aortic wall in ostial lesions.

❦ For "jailed" side-branch angioplasty, use only compliant balloons, which self-wrap after inflation and avoid the risk of entrapment.

❦ In stenting across side branch, choose a wire coil stent to ensure easy side branch access.

❦ Long lesion" definition:

- ≥10 mm (by CASS)
- 11 to 20 mm (newer definition)

❦ "Diffuse" disease implies lesions ≥20 mm in length or segments containing ≥3 discrete lesions.

❦ By AHA/ACC criteria, all lesions ≥20 mm long are type C lesions.

❦ Lesion length is an independent predictor of acute closure and restenosis.

❦ Rotablation offers the greatest benefits in long, eccentric, calcified, or ostial lesions; the restenosis rate remains still higher than for focal lesions.

❦ Technical considerations for long lesions:

- use long, noncompliant balloons
- use balloon:artery ratios of 1:1 rather than ≥1.1:1

❦ Regardless of the revascularization device used, the restenosis rate is higher for long lesions than for focal lesions.

❦ Angioplasty within the stents is safer than routine angioplasty.

❦ The coronary artery perforation is more frequent in elderly and in women.

❦ Patients suspected of possible perforation during revascularization are at risk of tamponade and should be observed in the hospital for ≥24 hours.

❦ The rate of perforation during high-pressure stent implantation is ~ 2%; in 90% of times it is evident at the time of angiography; in 10% of cases it may present as delayed cardiac tamponade.

❦ An occluded vessel with good collateral supply has the functional significance of 90% stenosis.

❦ The success rate for recanalization total occlusions is ~70%.

❦ The restenosis rate for total occlusions is 50% to 65%.

❦ TIMI grade flow ≥2 is a major predictor of survival and left ventricular function early and late after MI.

❦ The most frequent cause of failure to open a total occlusion is inability to cross with a guidewire.

❦ Total occlusions should be stented, as the rate of restenosis is lower in stented patients.

❦ Restenosis rate LAD< RCA<LCX (19%, 39%, 56%, respectively).

❦ *Ostial lesions* include the true ostium and the next 3 mm.

❦ Stenting of small vessels results in greater loss index and higher rates of cardiac events.

❦ Pathophysiology of SVG stenosis:

- <1 year: thrombus
- 1 to 5 years: IH
- >5 years: atherosclerosis

❦ *No reflow phenomenon* may result in piecemeal necrosis, rapid hemodynamic deterioration, and death.

❦ γ-Radiation therapy with ^{192}Ir reduced TVR by ~60% at 6 months (WRIST stent trial).

❦ Use of heparin-coated stents in acute MI resulted in

greater lumen diameter and lower restenosis and TVR rates at 6 months (STENT PAMI trial).

❦ The EPISTENT trial showed that *stenting plus abciximab* reduced the risk of death, MI, and vessel revascularization at 30-day and 6-month follow-up; reduction in death and MI was more prominent in patients with *unstable angina* within 48 hours; *diabetics* benefit as well, but they have worse outcomes than nondiabetics.

❦ Multivessel stenting is comparable with CABG for the composite endpoint of death, stroke, and MI; the rate of reinterventions was higher with stenting (ARTS trial).

❦ Use of oversized balloons (balloon:artery ratio ≥1.3) is a predictor of dissection, MI, and need for emergent surgery.

❦ Small edge dissections are not predictors of restenosis.

❦ SVG occlusion rates are 15% to 25% in the first post-operative year and 50% at 10 years.

❦ Distal embolization of atheromatous or thrombotic material occurs in 2% to 6% of cases of balloon angioplasty of SVGs.

❦ Restenosis rates are highest in aorto-ostial lesions, ranging from 56% to 80%.

❦ Stenting of de novo lesions of SVG is the considered the treatment of choice.

❦ TIMI 3 flow at 90 minutes is obtained in 30%, 50%, and 90% of patients treated with streptokinase, tPA, and primary angioplasty, respectively.

❦ Early reocclusion after thrombolysis occurs in 5% to 10% of patients, and late reocclusion in 30% to 40%.

❦ Primary PTCA for acute MI results in a 90% to 95% short-term patency and a 87% to 95% long-term patency.

❦ Stenting in acute MI is feasible and safe.

❦ *Bifurcation lesion* is defined as the presence of >50% stenosis within a main vessel and ostium of its side branch.

❦ Worsening of ostial stenosis (side branch) after stenting does not induce major clinical events in minor side branches (<2.5 mm).

❦ Revascularization of chronic total occlusions has both lower success rates and higher restenosis rates.

❦ Successful revascularization of chronic total occlusions is associated with improvement in anginal class and left ventricular function.

❦ Predictors of procedural success for total occlusions include age of the occlusion (75% <3 months and 37% >3 months), presence of antegrade flow (76% with and 58% without), angiographically tapered occlusion (77% versus 50%), absence of bridging collaterals (71% without versus 23% with), lesion length <15 mm, and absence of side branch.

❦ Aspirin reduces acute thrombotic complications during angioplasty.

❦ Dipyridamole does not convey any additional advantage when aspirin is being used during angioplasty.

❦ Aspirin plus ticlopidine is the regimen of choice when stenting is indicated.

❦ Ticlopidine after stenting for a total duration of 2 weeks appears to be as safe for 4 weeks and has a better safety profile.

❦ Additional antithrombotic regimens to aspirin and ticlopidine for patients at high risk for subacute thrombosis (major dissection, angiographic thrombus, abrupt closure, multiple stents, vessels <3 mm, or recent MI) are of unproven benefit.

❦ Abciximab, given as a bolus (0.25 m/kg) plus an infusion (10 μg/min), reduces acute and 6-month complications after angioplasty and after angioplasty plus stent.

❦ A lower heparin dose is used when abciximab is used, usually 70 U/kg bolus (maximum 7000 units) for a target ACT of 200 to 250.

❦ Pretreatment with heparin for >24 hours before angioplasty might provide a better angiographic and clinical success after angioplasty in high-risk patients (refractory unstable angina, I.C. thrombus).

❦ The HemoTec ACT test (Medtronic) yields values that are 30 to 50 seconds lower than those seen with the Hemochron (International Technidyne, Edison, NJ).

❦ It has not been proven that postprocedural heparin adds any benefit after angioplasty, even in high-risk patients or suboptimal results.

❧ Hirudin and bivalirudin (Hirulog; The Medicines Company, Cambridge, MA) are as efficacious as heparin during angioplasty.

❧ Thrombolytic therapy should not be routinely administered before angioplasty.

❧ Restenosis rarely presents as an acute coronary event (death or MI).

❧ Directional atherectomy does not reduce restenosis.

❧ β-Radiation penetrates only a few millimeters, can travel significant distances through air, can generate x-rays, and is not stopped by lead shielding.

❧ γ-Radiation requires strict radio protection.

❧ Percutaneous mitral valvuloplasty is indicated for symptomatic mitral stenosis, no recent embolic events, and no evidence of atrial thrombus by transesophageal ECHO and mitral insufficiency <2+.

❧ In Roto cases, avoid placing the wire in small branches or allowing looping of the wire.

❧ Maintain the burr speed within 5000 rpm of the platform speed.

❧ *Lame's equation* states that tension in a pressurized cylinder is proportional to the lumen size and inversely proportional to the thickness of the wall.

❧ Predictors of success for percutaneous mitral valvuloplasty include: balloon size, low ECHO score, younger age, normal sinus rhythm, NYHA Class I or II, no mitral insufficiency, and fluoroscopic degree of calcification.

❧ Balloon pulmonic valvuloplasty is indicated for symptomatic pulmonary valvular stenosis, or asymptomatic with a gradient >80 mm Hg and no evidence of severe pulmonic insufficiency, associated subvalvular stenosis and severe pulmonary annular hypoplasia.

❧ Vessel diameter is estimated by comparing it with the guiding catheter: **1F = 0.33 mm.**

❧ Eccentric lesions should not be treated primarily with rotablation unless IVUS shows significant calcification.

❧ *Dotter effect:* the more severe the lesion, the higher the gain in MLD.

❧ For rotablation cases, use temporary pacemaker for RCA, dominant circumflex, ostial LAD, and burrs ≥2.25 mm.

❧ Regarding multivessel PTCA versus CABG in nondiabetic patients, mortality rates were shown to be the same; the in-hospital rate of acute MI was higher for the surgical approach.

❧ Patients with single vessel disease and poor left ventricular function have worse prognosis than patients with 3-vessel disease and normal left ventricular function.

❧ *Complete revascularization* is better than incomplete revascularization, regardless of the mode of revascularization.

❧ Incomplete revascularization is acceptable when a vessel is too small to be bypassed (≤1.5 mm) or serves a nonviable territory.

❧ In multivessel PTCA, start with the vessel supplying the largest jeopardized area.

❧ To prevent balloon entrapment in the implanted stent, only compliant (self-wrapping) balloons should be used to dilate side branches.

❧ "T stenting" for trunk vessel-side branch is associated with higher complication rates compared with stenting the trunk vessel and only dilating the side branch.

❧ A CFR ≥2.5 after PTCA predicts good clinical outcome, low risk of immediate complications, and low restenosis rate.

❧ There is a dose response for radiation; most studies suggest a minimum effective dose of 15 Gy at the source.

❧ Brachytherapy reduces stent restenosis.

❧ Radioactive stents are associated with a "candy wrapper" effect more commonly than I.C. radiation.

❧ Stents are the preferable initial choice for vessels larger than 3.0 mm.

❧ IVUS is indicated in the evaluation of post-cardiac-transplantation patients undergoing coronary angiography.

❧ CFR <2.0 is associated with a positive stress test.

❦ FFR <0.75 is associated with ischemia.

❦ CFR <2.0 after balloon angioplasty should receive a stent if feasible.

❦ FFR <0.9 and >0.75 after balloon angioplasty should be considered for stenting.

❦ Bifurcational lesions should be treated with debulking therapy, followed by main vessel stenting and balloon angioplasty of the side branch.

❦ Intra-vein-graft injection of verapamil (100 μg) before angioplasty/primary stenting might reduce the no reflow rates.

❦ Dissections that do not produce pressure gradient or generate a CFR >2.0, large lumen, and normal distal flow do not necessarily require stent placement.

❦ "T stent" restenosis is very high (up to 70%, with 40% involving both branches).

❦ The restenosis rate for stents is approximately 1.07% × mm of stented vessel.

Classification of Coronary Artery Perforations

Type of Perforation	Description	Treatment
Type I	Extraluminal crater, no extravasation	Prolonged inflations with perfusion balloons; can continue aspirin, heparin
Type II	Pericardial/myocardial blush, no extravasation	The same as type I, 2-D ECHO
Type III	Extravasation through frank perforation ("jet extravasation")	2-D ECHO "stat" to r/o pericardial effusion; protamine to reverse anticoagulation; endoluminal grafts (covered stents)
Cavity Spilling	Perforation into a cardiac chamber, coronary sinus	The same as type III

- Rate of perforation:
    0.1% - PTCA (use balloon-to-artery ratio ≤1.1)
    0.5% to 3% - TEC, DCA, ELCA (use device-to artery ratio ≤0.8)
- Steps to be taken in case of perforation:
    1. Notify cardiac surgeons and have OR ready.
    2. Inflate a balloon at 2 to 6 atm for ≥ 10 minutes balloon-to-artery ratio 0.9 to 1.0)
    3. If sealing incomplete, use a perfusion balloon at low pressure for 15 to 45 min; flush the lumen intermittently with heparinized saline. Prolonged balloon inflations are successful in 60% to 70% of perforations.
    4. If sealing not successful, start giving protamine in incremental doses (25 to 50 mg over 10 to 30 minutes)
    5. ECHO
    6. If pericardial effusion is present, insert a multiple-sidehole catheter in pericardial space.
    7. Emergency surgery is required in 30% to 40% of coronary artery perforations.

Time After CABG and Location of the SVG Lesion Influence the Rate of Restenosis After PTCA

Time After CABG/Location	Restenosis Rate After PTCA
≤1 year	≤45%
≥1 year	≥60%
Proximal and mid vein graft	60% to 70%
Distal anastomotic	45%

Angioplasty of a proximal anastomotic segment of a degenerating 10-year-old graft has poor long-term success.

NHLBI Classification of Coronary Artery Dissections

Dissection Type	Description
A	Minimal radiolucency, not persistent
B	**"Double lumen,"** not persistent
C	**Extraluminal cap** with persistence of contrast dye after the lumen cleared
D	**Spiral**
E	Persistent, new filling defect
F	Dissection resulting in impaired flow/total occlusion

- Types A and B do not increase the risk of acute closure.
- Types C through F are associated with a 5-fold risk of MI, emergency CABG, and death.
- Complex dissections contain deep medial tears.
- Complex dissection is the most powerful predictor of acute closure.

Abbreviations Used in this Book

ABI = ankle-brachial index
ABSI = ankle/brachial systolic index
ACC = American College of Cardiology
ACP = American College of Physicians
ACT = activated clotting time
ADP = adenosine diphosphate
aPTT = activated partial thromboplastin time
APV = average peak velocity
A/T = aspirin/ticlopidine
AT III = antithrombin III
AV = atrioventricular
AVG-LCX = atrioventricular groove-left circumflex
A/W = aspirin/warfarin
BP = blood pressure
Ca^{++} = intracellular calcium
CABG = coronary artery bypass graft
CAD = coronary artery disease
cAMP = cyclic 3′, 5′-adenosine monophosphate
CCU = critical care unit
C/E = cost-effectiveness (ratio)
CFR = coronary flow reserve
CFVR = coronary flow velocity reserve
cGMP = cyclic (3′, 5′-) guanosine monophosphate
CHF = congestive heart failure
CK-MB = creatine kinase MB band
CMV = cytomegalovirus
COPD = chronic obstructive pulmonary disease
CPK = creatine phosphokinase
CSA = cross-sectional area
CTFC = corrected TIMI frame count

CVA = cerebrovascular accident
DCA = directional coronary atherectomy
ECG = electrocardiogram
ECHO = echocardiogram
EDTA = edetic acid
EECP = external enhanced counterpulsation
ELCA = excimer laser coronary angioplasty
FDA = Food and Drug Administration
FFR = fractional flow reserve
FFRmyo = fractional flow reserve of the myocardium
Gp IIb/IIIa = glycoprotein IIb/IIIa
GTP = guanosine triphosphate
HACA = human antichimeric antibody
HDL = high-density lipoprotein
HIT = heparin-induced thrombocytopenia
HR = heart rate
I.C. = intracoronary
IH = intimal hyperplasia
IMA = internal mammary artery
INR = international normalized ratio
IU = international unit
I.V. = intravenous
IVUS = intravascular ultrasound
LAD = left anterior descending (coronary artery)
LAO = left anterior oblique
LBBB = left bundle branch block
LCA = left coronary artery
LCX = left circumflex (coronary artery)
LDL = low-density lipoprotein
LDH = lactic dehydrogenase
LIMA = left IMA
LM = left main (coronary artery)
LMWH = low molecular weight heparin
MI = myocardial infarction
MLD = minimum luminal diameter
Na^+/H^+ = sodium/hydrogen exchange
NCRP = National Council on Radiation Protection
NHLBI = National Heart, Lung, and Blood Institute
NO = nitric oxide
NPH = neutral protamine Hagedorn
OR = operating room
PCI = percutaneous coronary intervention

PDA = posterior descending (coronary) artery
PET = positron-emission tomography
PG = prostaglandin
PGI_2 = prostacyclin
P.O. = by mouth
POBA = plain old balloon angioplasty
PT = prothrombin time
PTCA = percutaneous transluminal coronary angioplasty
Q = every
QALY = quality-adjusted life year
QD = every day
RAO = right anterior oblique
RCA = right coronary artery
SAM = surface-adherent monocyte
S.L. = sublingual
S.Q. = subcutaneous
SVG = saphenous vein graft
TEC = transluminal extraction catheter
TIMI = thrombolysis in myocardial infarction
TMR = transmyocardial laser revascularization
tPA = tissue plasminogen activator
TTP = thrombotic thrombocytopenic purpura
U = unit
XB and EBU = extra back-up